Ride List

DISCLAIMER

This book is meant only as a guide to select road rides within Los Angeles County and does not guarantee rider safety in any way—have fun but know you ride at your own risk. Neither Menasha Ridge Press nor Patrick Brady is liable for property loss or damage, personal injury, or death that results in any way from accessing or riding the routes described in the following pages. Be especially cautious when riding down steep roads. Be vigilant regarding motorized vehicles and other cyclists—especially when on group rides. To help ensure an uneventful ride, please read carefully the introduction to this book. Familiarize yourself thoroughly with the areas you intend to visit before venturing out. Ask questions, and prepare for the unforeseen. Familiarize yourself with current weather reports and maps of the area you intend to visit, and observe all road regulations.

Copyright © 2007 by Patrick Brady

All rights reserved
Published by Menasha Ridge Press
Printed in the United States of America
Distributed by Publishers Group West
First edition, first printing

Text and cover design by Alian Design
Cover photograph by Patrick Brady
Author photograph by Greg Page
All other photographs by Patrick Brady
Cartography and elevation profiles by Patrick Brady, Chris Erichson, and
    Scott McGrew

Brady, Patrick, 1963–
    Bicycling Los Angeles County : a guide to great road bike rides /
    Patrick Brady. — 1st ed.
        p. cm.
    Includes bibliographical references and index.
    ISBN-13: 978-0-89732-950-7 (alk. paper)
    ISBN-10: 0-89732-950-3 (alk. paper)
    1. Cycling—California—Los Angeles County—Guidebooks. 2. Bicycle trails—
        California—Los Angeles County—Guidebooks. 3. Bicycle touring—
        California—Los Angeles County—Guidebooks. 4. Los Angeles County
        (Calif.)—Guidebooks. I. Title.
    GV1045.5.C22B73 2007
    791.06'80979493--dc22

                            2007026133

Menasha Ridge Press
P.O. Box 43673
Birmingham, AL 35243
www.menasharidge.com

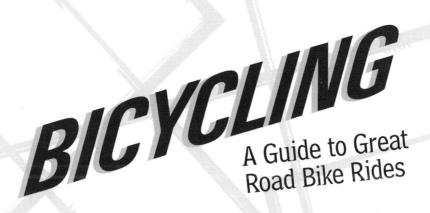

BICYCLING

A Guide to Great
Road Bike Rides

Los Angeles County

Patrick Brady

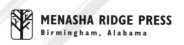

MENASHA RIDGE PRESS
Birmingham, Alabama

Contents

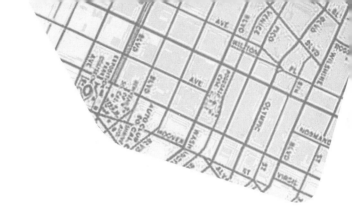

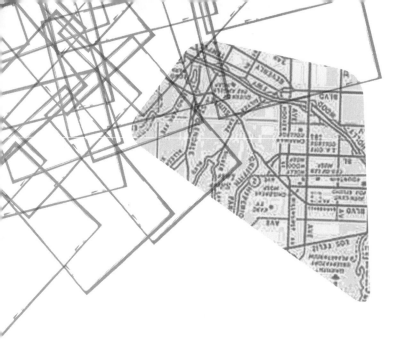

I dedicate this book to my family. My parents, Gabriel Brady and Kathryn Vowell, my stepparents, Lei Brady and Byron Vowell, and my sister, Erin Kathleen, have shown unflinching belief in me, and for that I am forever grateful.

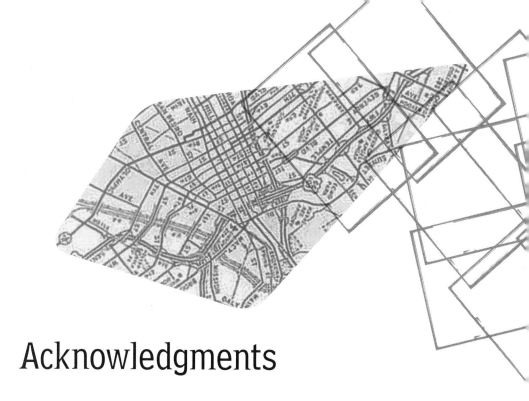

Acknowledgments

A number of people made significant contributions to this book. When I undertook the project, I can't really say I appreciated just how much the kindness of friends would matter. Everyone who joined me for one of the rides (and put up with my stopping to set a waypoint or take a photo) gets a special nod. Through the years, many people inspired my curiosity about new roads here in Los Angeles. Among these folks: Lorraine Daly, Jeff Dykzeul, Phil Carter, Kevin Philips, and Ron Peterson. Banner Moffatt and Mimi Sheean proved to be valuable resources for the insider's scoop on the Montrose Ride. Without their assistance, my description of the ride(s) wouldn't have been as accurate. My editor,

Russell Helms, has been a great support through this process, providing guidance, praise, and valued friendship. Greg Page deserves greater appreciation and credit than I can demonstrate in this space. His advice on routes, tips on taking even better photos, unfailing friendship, and companionship for many of these rides may never be adequately rewarded. Finally, I save my greatest praise for my girlfriend, Shana Reid, for her patience, her belief in my abilities, her eternal curiosity, and her willingness to drive support for me on one very long day in the saddle. With her sunny disposition, she can make a trip to the stockyards a good time, and a fun day in the mountains mythic.

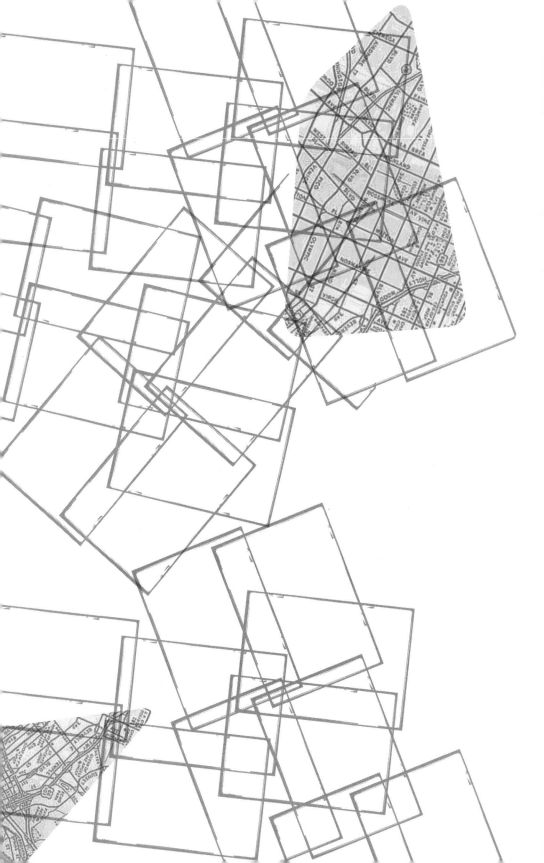

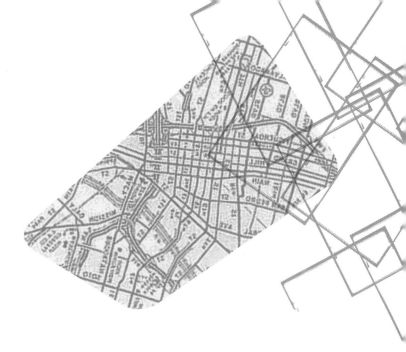

Preface

Since the age of six, when I outpedaled the babysitter who was acting as my training wheels, the bicycle has been one of my favorite expressions of freedom. Any time I look at a map, I see a point of convergence involving me, my bicycle, the future, and fun. In my life, the bicycle has served as a great deal more than just exercise or transportation. It's the source of my social life, many of my peak experiences as a human being, and much of my mental health. The simple fact is, I love cycling as much today as I did when I was six.

In early 1996, I was a freelance writer living in Northampton, Massachusetts, which is in the Pioneer Valley, an area considered by almost anyone who has ever lived there to be a little slice of heaven. I spent my summers road riding, mountain biking, and inline skating. And I spent my winters cross-country and downhill skiing; I was even an instructor in cross-country skiing at a local ski area.

I wasn't making much of a living, though. And when a chance emerged to move to Los Angeles to join the staff of *Bicycle Guide* magazine, I leapt. Arguably one of the most respected cycling magazines ever published, *BG* was known for high editorial standards, and its editors had a reputation for being both knowledgable and fit. The friend and University of Massachusetts, Amherst cycling teammate who recommended me for the gig, a current *Bicycling* contributing editor named Alan Coté, lamented that I'd be moving to the "on-ramp to the apocalypse." I reminded him that I had grown up in the Deep South (without mountains or coastline, the Mississippi Delta isn't my idea of pretty) and went on to say that I believed I could find plenty to enjoy in the greater Los Angeles metropolis. Boy, was I right. Living in Los Angeles has been an odyssey. I've lived all over—the West Side, the Santa Clarita Valley, and the South Bay. Each has its charms.

As a staffer for *BG,* I endeavored to learn about the rides and races around the area. I joined a variety of clubs, drove to races several area codes away, and branched out on my own from time to time. The fact is, I've been a student ever since.

In 2002, after many fits and starts, I launched *Asphalt Magazine,* a road-cycling publication aimed at the dedicated cycling enthusiast. I believed that there was a need for a journal that spoke to hard-core roadies. *Asphalt* was praised for its high editorial and print standards and enjoyed enthusiastic support from its readers and the industry. Unfortunately, the abrupt departure of my partner doomed the magazine.

In promoting *Asphalt,* I traveled to many different group rides in LA and Orange County. The incredible variety of riding conditions and climatic variation has never ceased to amaze me. However, *Asphalt* ceased publication before I had a chance to do a feature on the range of riding here. That desire has been nagging at me until now.

People talk of the incredible riding in the Bay Area. San Francisco has a much better reputation as a place to enjoy cycling than Los Angeles does. A friend, the noted cycling author and Marin County resident Owen Mulholland, lends his considerable intellect to the task of pitying my predicament (suffering the ills of LA) whenever we are on the phone. Frankly, this is my chance to set the record straight.

It's true that the cost of living and traffic can make life in Los Angeles difficult and frustrating. However, it hasn't been so bad to cause me to consider moving away, at least, not more seriously than as an idle fantasy. My typical Sunday ride meets in Manhattan Beach and heads to Malibu, where we ascend Topanga Canyon Road, bomb down to Mulholland, and climb Piuma or Stunt before the drop to the beach and the flat return home. There's a turnout on Piuma (marked as a waypoint in this guide) with a view of the mountains rushing headlong into the ocean that is of such breathtaking grandeur and sweeping drama that I am reminded how grateful I am to be alive. I'm also lucky to enjoy such beauty on a routine basis.

I've ridden all over the United States and led bicycle tours in the Alps, the Pyrenees, Provence, and Tuscany. In terms of visual beauty, the challenge of the terrain, and the sheer fun of the descents, Malibu (and, for that matter, Palos Verdes) is a match for any of them.

Lest someone think I've been smoking something illicit, I must admit that this "city" isn't a friendly place for bicycle commuters. There are areas of LA that I simply won't ride in or through. I've worked all over and, although I have commuted to work by bicycle at a few jobs, for most of those places riding a bike simply hasn't been a realistic possibility. LA has some fascinating places rich in history or scenic value that, because of traffic or the neighborhood, don't make the list of smart places to bike. After a good deal of research, I came to the conclusion that some locations were a little too sketchy— even at 7 a.m. on a Saturday or Sunday morning—to suggest a route there.

Many of these rides suggest an early start, often on a weekend day. I do not make these recommendations lightly. These routes should not be attempted on weekdays, especially during morning or afternoon rush hours—at least not unless you were raised by bike messengers or grizzly bears ... preferably both.

For the sake of simplicity, all the rides in this guide are loops of one form or another. There isn't a ride here that requires shuttling, which would necessitate the assistance of a friend or family member.

While you may need to drive to the start of the ride, you won't need another car to get back to the start, ever.

This guide offers a significant variation from its predecessors and competition in that it offers details on some of LA's group rides. My purpose in doing this was twofold—to offer local riders the opportunity to try new and challenging routes against the best legs in that area, and to give visiting riders an instant well of opportunity.

Whenever I travel, I try to bring my bike with me, and I always contact a club before my arrival to inquire about the weekend group rides. Without fail, the strategy has resulted in new friendships, fun rides, and exposure to roads I might not have noticed on a map. A guidebook of this sort would have saved me a lot of work. Honestly, part of the fun of a group ride is not having to stop to check where the turn is and instead zoom through it.

Bicycle clubs populate Los Angeles (seemingly) everywhere the gangs do not. There are literally dozens of clubs, and each has its own rides. There are more of these rides than I could hope to include in any one book. In order to choose which rides I would include, I established some guidelines. First, the ride has to recur each week on the same day and the same route. That rendered ineligible a great many rides because most clubs vary their rides from week to week. Indeed, many hold meetings in which members choose among their favorite rides to include them in the rotation. Finally, I'm not much of a party crasher, and I wanted wherever possible to include rides that drew riders from the region, rather than from just the nearest club.

There is one notable exception to my criteria: the Simi Ride. The ride is seasonal (it's too hot to try this ride in July), and the course varies from early fall until late winter, when its members return to racing; also, much of the ride is in Ventura County. That said, the ride is arguably one of the most famous group rides anywhere. There isn't an aspiring Category IV racer in Los Angeles who hasn't shown his cards at the Simi Ride.

In writing this guide, I endeavored to offer something for everyone, from those looking for new places to take a spin on their beach cruisers to devout roadies who want to try new group rides. Not every ride in this guide will suit every reader, but I guarantee there is a ride to suit everyone who rides a bike. Have fun out there.

In writing this guide, I endeavored to offer something for everyone, from those looking for new places to take a spin on their beach cruisers to devout roadies who want to try new group rides.

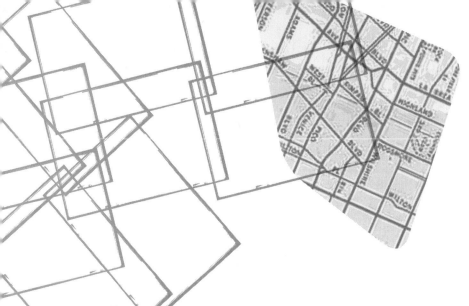

Introduction:
How to Use This Guidebook

The Overview Map and Overview-Map Key
Use the overview map on the inside front cover to assess the location of each ride's primary trailhead. Each ride's number appears on the overview map, on the map key facing the overview map, in the table of contents, and at the top of the ride description's pages.

Trail Maps
Each ride contains a detailed map that shows the trailhead, the route, significant features, facilities, and topographic landmarks such as creeks, overlooks, and peaks. The author gathered map data by carrying a Garmin eTrex Legend GPS unit while riding. GPS data was downloaded into a digital mapping program, DeLorme Topo USA, and processed by expert cartographers to produce the highly accurate maps found in this book. Each trailhead's GPS coordinates are included with each profile (see page xiii).

Elevation Profiles
Corresponding directly to the trail map, a detailed elevation profile is given for each ride. The elevation profile provides a quick look at the trail from the side, enabling you to visualize how it rises and falls. Note the number of feet between each tick mark on the vertical axis (the height scale). To avoid making flat rides look steep and steep rides appear flat, appropriate height scales are used throughout the book to provide an accurate image of each ride's climbing difficulty. Elevation profiles for loop rides show total distance; those for out-and-back rides show only one-way distance.

GPS Trailhead Coordinates
In addition to GPS-based maps, this book also includes the GPS coordinates for each trailhead in two formats: latitude-longitude and UTM (Universal Transverse Mercator). Latitude-longitude coordinates employ a grid system that indicates your location by crossroading a line that runs north to south

with a line that runs east to west. Lines of latitude are parallel and run east to west; the 0° line of latitude is the equator. Lines of longitude are not parallel, run north to south, and converge at the North and South poles; the 0° line of longitude passes through Greenwich, England.

Topographic maps show latitude and longitude in addition to UTM grid lines. Known as UTM coordinates, the numbers index a specific Earth point, also using a grid method. The survey information, or datum, used to arrive at the coordinates in this book is WGS84 (versus NAD27 or WGS83). For readers who own a GPS unit, whether handheld or onboard a vehicle, the latitude–longitude or UTM coordinates provided on the first page of each ride may be entered into the GPS unit. Just make sure your GPS unit is set to navigate using WGS84 datum. Now you can navigate directly to the trailhead.

Trailheads in parking areas can be reached by car, but some rides still require a short walk or ride to reach the official trailhead from the parking area. In those cases, a handheld unit is necessary to continue the GPS-navigation process. That said, readers can easily access all trailheads in this book without a GPS unit by using the directions given, the overview maps, and the trail maps, which show at least one significant road leading into the area. But for those who enjoy using the latest GPS technology to navigate, the necessary data have been provided. A brief explanation of the UTM coordinates for Topanga Canyon Loop (page 8) follows.

UTM Zone	11S
Easting	361717
Northing	3764453

The UTM Zone number 11 refers to one of the 60 vertical zones of the UTM projection, each of which is 6 degrees wide. The "S"

refers to horizontal zones, each of which is 8 degrees wide, except for Zone X (12 degrees wide). The easting number, 361717, indicates in meters how far east or west a point is from the central meridian of the zone. Increasing easting coordinates on a topographic map or on your GPS screen indicate that you are moving east; decreasing easting coordinates indicate that you are moving west. The northing number, 3764453, references in meters how far you are from the equator. Increasing northing coordinates indicate you are traveling north; decreasing northing coordinates indicate you are traveling south. To learn more about how to enhance your outdoor experiences with GPS technology, refer to *GPS Outdoors: A Practical Guide for Outdoor Enthusiasts* (Menasha Ridge Press).

Ride Description

Each ride contains a detailed description of the route from beginning to end. The description is the heart of each ride. Here, the author provides a summary of the trail's essence and highlights any extras the ride has to offer. The route is clearly outlined, including landmarks, side trips, and possible alternate routes along the way. The main narrative is enhanced with an "In Brief" description of the ride, a Key At-a-Glance Information box, and driving directions to the trailhead. Many rides include a note on nearby activities, such as where to grab a cold brew after the ride.

IN BRIEF

A "taste of the ride." Think of this section as a snapshot focused on the historic landmarks, scenic vistas, and other sights you may encounter on the ride.

KEY AT-A-GLANCE INFORMATION

The information in the Key At-a-Glance boxes gives you quick statistics and specifics for each ride.

Length: The length of the ride from start to finish (total distance traveled). There may be options to shorten or extend the ride, but the mileage corresponds to the described ride. Consult the ride description for help deciding how to customize the ride for your ability or time constraints.

Configuration: A description of what the ride might look like from overhead. Rides can be loops, out-and-backs, figure-eights, or a combination of shapes.

Aerobic Difficulty: On average, how out of breath you can expect to be; the scale ranges from 1 (supereasy) to 5 (bring bottled oxygen).

Technical Difficulty: On average, how tricky a particular ride is to negotiate because of terrain, traffic, and other variables; the scale ranges from 1 (look, no hands!) to 5 (bring the training wheels).

Scenery: A short summary of what to expect in terms of plant life, wildlife, natural wonders, and historic features.

Exposure: A quick check of how much sun you can expect on your shoulders during the ride.

Ride Traffic: Indicates how busy the ride might be on an average day. Traffic, of course, varies from day to day and season to season.

Trail Surface: Indicates any surfaces other than smooth asphalt that you may encounter.

Riding Time: The length of time it takes to complete the ride. For these rides, I assume an average speed of 15 mph—very reasonable for a short, flat route, but a fairly strenuous workout for the more mountainous rides.

Access: A notation of any fees or permits that may be needed to access the trail or park at the trailhead.

Maps: The name(s) of relevant USGS topo maps and/or maps available at trailheads.

Facilities: What to expect in terms of restrooms and water at the trailhead or key stops along the way.

DIRECTIONS
Used in conjunction with the overview map, the driving directions lead you to the trailhead. Once at the trailhead, park only in designated areas.

Weather
Southern California may benefit from an enviable climate relative to the rest of the United States, but Los Angeles is a varied place, climatically speaking. During the winter, differences in temperature between coastal areas and the inland basin and valleys will be slight. But in the summer, the cool Alaska current keeps temperatures at the coast very moderate, while the valleys bake—temperatures routinely exceed 100°F from July to September.

Rainfall is typically infrequent in Los Angeles County, except during the winter, when the average number of days with rainfall climbs to seven for the season. It's not a great idea to ride during or just following rain; because rain is rare, when it does come, accumulated oil on the streets makes them unusually hazardous for cyclists.

Though it isn't generally publicized, the coast does experience a fair amount of fog. The Beach Cities (Manhattan Beach, Hermosa Beach, and Redondo Beach) and the Palos Verdes Peninsula experience a great deal of morning fog during the summer. Morning and afternoon temperatures can also be suppressed by the marine layer—low-lying cloud cover that isn't quite low enough to count as fog.

THE COAST
AVERAGE TEMPERATURES BY MONTH
(FAHRENHEIT)

Jan	Feb	Mar	Apr	May	Jun
HIGH					
64°	64°	64°	65°	66°	69°
LOW					
45°	45°	46°	48°	51°	54°

Jul	Aug	Sep	Oct	Nov	Dec
HIGH					
71°	73°	73°	71°	69°	65°
LOW					
57°	59°	57°	53°	48°	45°

INLAND CITIES AND VALLEYS
AVERAGE TEMPERATURES BY MONTH
(FAHRENHEIT)

Jan	Feb	Mar	Apr	May	Jun
HIGH					
64°	64°	64°	65°	66°	69°
LOW					
45°	45°	46°	48°	51°	54°

Jul	Aug	Sep	Oct	Nov	Dec
HIGH					
71°	73°	73°	71°	69°	65°
LOW					
57°	59°	57°	53°	48°	45°

Because of the area's stellar climate, you can enjoy cycling in Los Angeles year-round. Indeed, the only time one might rule out riding would be in the mid- to late afternoons in the valleys during the summer.

Water
Always err on the side of excess when deciding how much water or electrolyte-based sports drinks to pack: A rider working hard in 90°F heat needs about 10 quarts of fluid per day; that's about 2.5 gallons. In other words, pack along one or two bottles, even for short rides. For long rides, especially in hot weather, consider cameling water on your back in a hydration system.

While some of the rides contained in this guide are long and ambitious, riders are never more than an hour from a convenience store. Armed with a few bucks and two 24-ounce bottles, you will be able to stay properly hydrated on even the hottest days in the desert.

Clothing
Most of these rides can be completed in shorts and a short-sleeved jersey. Cooler conditions usually call for the addition of only a base layer, vest, long-finger gloves, arm warmers, and knee warmers. During the months of December and January, the early-morning group rides might call for something a little heavier—full tights, a jacket, toe covers, and maybe a skullcap. Truly, the only real mistake you can make is to overdress on a cold morning; it always warms up. Stick with layers and small items that can be removed.

The Essentials
One of the first rules of riding is to be prepared for anything. The simplest way to be prepared is to carry the essentials. In addition to carrying the items listed on the next page, you need to know how to use them, especially the navigation items. Always consider worst-case scenarios, such as getting lost, riding back in the dark, breaking components, crashing, or encountering a brutal thunderstorm. The items listed below don't cost a lot of money, don't take up much

room in a pack, and don't weigh much—but they might just save your life.

1. water: durable bottles

2. map: preferably a topo map and a copy of this book's trail map and ride description

3. GPS unit

4. first-aid kit: a compact, high-quality kit including first-aid instructions

5. knife: a bike multitool with a knife is best

6. extra food: you should always have some left when you've finished riding

7. extra clothes: rain protection, warm layers, gloves, warm hat

8. sun protection: sunglasses, lip balm, sunblock, sun hat (in case you have to walk)

9. cell phone: you will have coverage in most areas

Topo Maps

The maps in this book have been produced with great care and, used with the directions, will direct you to the trail and help you stay on course. However, you will find additional detail and valuable information in the United States Geological Survey's 7.5-minute series topographic maps. Topo maps are available online in many locations. The downside to USGS topos is that many of them are outdated, having been created 20 to 30 years ago. Cultural features on outdated topo maps, such as roads, will probably be inaccurate, but the topographic features should be accurate.

Digital topographic-map programs such as DeLorme's TopoUSA enable you to review topo maps of the entire United States on your PC; gathered while hiking with a GPS unit, data can be downloaded onto the software so you can plot your own rides. And Google Earth is a great free program that allows you to check aerial views of an area against a topo map.

If you're new to maps, you might be wondering what a topo map is. In short, a topo map indicates not only linear distance but elevation as well, using contour lines. Each brown squiggly line represents a particular elevation, and at the base of each topo a contour's interval designation is given. If the contour interval is 20 feet, then the distance between each contour line is 20 feet. Follow five contour lines up on the same map, and the elevation has increased by 100 feet. Every fifth contour line is labeled with an altitude. These lines are slightly heavier than the intervening contour lines and are called the index lines. An index line that reads "1,300" indicates a contour that is 1,300 feet above sea level.

In addition to the outdoor shops listed in the Appendixes, you'll find topos at major universities and some public libraries, where you can photocopy the maps you need and save yourself buying them. But if you want your own and can't find them locally, visit the USGS's Web site at topomaps.usgs.gov.

Also, don't overlook locally produced maps, which usually show superior detail for small areas. Examples include county road maps. Another reliable map source that contains updated road information on topo maps is DeLorme's *Gazetteer* series. There is a *Gazetteer* for each of the 50 states.

Bike Tools

Even for short rides, carrying these basics requires only a small seat bag. The most common problem is probably the dreaded flat. If you opt for carrying only compressed air to re-inflate tires, you run the risk of having more flats than you have air cylinders; a small frame pump solves that problem. Before you go, make sure your tire-patch kit's rubber cement hasn't dried out. Also, if your chain snaps, you'll need a chain tool to piece it back together (and for Shimano chains, you'll need a replacement pin as well). Here is a complete list of the tools you'll need:

1. spare tube
2. patch kit
3. frame pump and/or CO_2 cartridges
4. tire levers
5. chain tool
6. multitool
7. cell phone

The multitool should address the balance of repairs or adjustments (e.g., to seat, brakes, derailleurs) you may need to make on a ride. If an accident necessitates more serious repairs, well, that's what the cell phone is for.

First-Aid Kit
A very basic first-aid kit may contain more items than you might think necessary. Prepackaged kits in waterproof bags are available (Atwater Carey and Adventure Medical make a variety of kits). Though there are quite a few items listed here, they pack into a small space:

- Antibiotic ointment (Neosporin or the generic equivalent) for cuts
- Aspirin or acetaminophen for aches
- Band-Aids for cuts
- Benadryl or the generic equivalent, diphenhydramine (in case of allergic reactions)
- Butterfly-closure bandages for deep cuts
- Epinephrine in a prefilled syringe (for people known to have severe allergic reactions to such things as bee stings)

General Safety
Potentially dangerous situations can occur, but preparation and sound judgment result in safe forays into remote and wild areas. Here are a few tips to make your trip safer and easier:

- Always carry food and water.
- Wear sturdy cycling shoes.
- Wear an American National Standards Institute–approved cycling helmet.
- Never ride alone—take a buddy with you or join a group ride.
- Tell someone where you're going and when you'll be back (be as specific as possible), and ask him or her to get help if you don't return in a reasonable amount of time.
- Stay on the routes described herein. Most riders get lost when they leave the planned route.
- Take along your brain. A cool, calculating mind is the single most important piece of equipment you'll need on the road. Think before you act. Watch your self. Plan ahead. Avoiding accidents before they happen is the best strategy for a rewarding and relaxing ride.

Hazards
For the most part, road conditions on each of these rides are excellent. One will occasionally encounter a pothole or other unruly pavement, but most streets are swept weekly, so debris doesn't tend to build up. The greatest ongoing hazard in Southern California comes from traffic. Los Angeles is ruled by the automobile. Most of the roads navigated in this guide are more lightly traveled than LA's most heavily driven

thoroughfares. There are some exceptions; in these instances, start your ride as early as is practical and, if possible, do theride on a weekend day. Saturday and Sunday mornings are more conducive to safe cycling than are any other times of the week.

All this traffic leads to another eventuality: parked cars. Getting doored (having a driver of a parked car open the door into your path) can have mortal consequences here. Maintain a good lookout of what's going on in the parked cars to your right, and leave yourself some room to maneuver, if possible.

The mountain routes contained in this guide include some roads that occasionally experience rockfall. Exercise caution on the descents because it is possible to find material spilling into the road. Also, some of the mountain roads in Malibu include off-camber turns and turns that decrease in radius as you follow the road. Exercise restraint the first time you freewheel down any of these roads.

Road Etiquette

Treat motorists, fellow riders, and others with respect. Bicyclists have every right to ride on area roads, with the exception of interstates. Just remember that motorists may not be aware of your right to share the road. Motorists may also be unfamiliar with bicycling signals and navigation techniques. Avoid confrontation with motorists and always attempt to crush rudeness with kindness. Do not, though, compromise your safety in any way. Ultimately, do what it takes to stay safe. Here are a few more tips to stay safe and end the day with a grin:

- Respect road closures (ask if not sure) and avoid trespassing on private land.
- Indicate your intentions. Even using the most rudimentary hand signals increases your safety by telling drivers what you plan to do.
- Do not litter. No one likes to see the trash someone else has left behind.
- Plan ahead. Know your bike, your ability, and the area in which you are riding—and prepare accordingly. Be self-sufficient at all times; carry necessary supplies for changes in weather or other conditions.

> # Treat motorists, fellow riders, and others with respect. Bicyclists have every right to ride on area roads, with the exception of interstates.

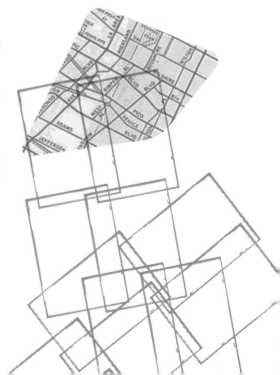

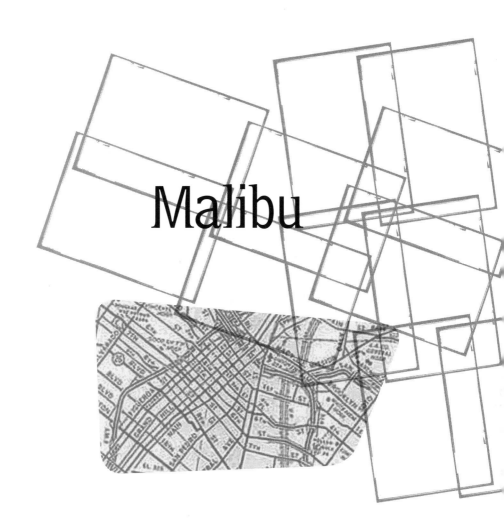

Malibu

1 Mulholland Highway Loop

AT A GLANCE

Length: 72 miles

Configuration: Loop

Difficulty: Difficult

Climbing: 5,000 feet

Maximum gradient: 13%

Scenery: Ocean, canyons, vineyards, and the Los Angeles coastline

Exposure: Usually sunny; can be overcast in winter

Road traffic: Pacific Coast Highway is busy, but otherwise traffic is pretty light

Road surface: Generally good, though there can be occasional rockfall resulting in some gravel near canyon walls

Riding time: 5 hours

Maps: Los Angeles County *Thomas Guide* pages 671, 631, 630, 629, 628, 668, 667, 627, 626, 625, 586, 587, 588, 589, and 590

In Brief

The canyon roads of Malibu haven't got the reputation of its surf, but they ought to. These asphalt ribbons have it all: steep pitches, dramatic vistas, technical turns, and sweeping, no-brake descents. This is arguably some of the finest riding in the world. These canyon roads are popular not only with cyclists but also with motorcyclists and sports car enthusiasts. The two climbs will take you above 2,000 feet elevation, making this one of the tougher routes in this book. That said, this ride is worth every drop of sweat you'll surrender; the views are truly world class.

Directions

This ride begins in Santa Monica at the world-famous Santa Monica Pier. Parking is inexpensive and plentiful, provided you arrive in the morning. To get to the pier, travel west on I-10 from I-405. Exit the 10 at Fourth Street and shift into the left lane.

Turn left at Colorado Avenue and proceed south two blocks and turn right on Seaside Terrace. You will immediately see signs for parking. Free street parking isn't easy to find nearby.

Description

Like many rides in this book, because of the nature of Los Angeles traffic, this loop is easier and safer if you ride it in the morning. Easier because the heat will be less, and safer because the outbound ride goes against the morning traffic that's heading into Los Angeles. Weekend mornings are preferable to weekday mornings, though the latter can be good if you start the ride following rush hour, which ends around 9 a.m.

The ride begins on the beach bike path that skirts the parking lot on its west and north sides. Ride north (the ocean will be to your left) on the bike path for 2.9 miles. When you reach the parking lot at Temescal Canyon Road, exit the bike path and turn left

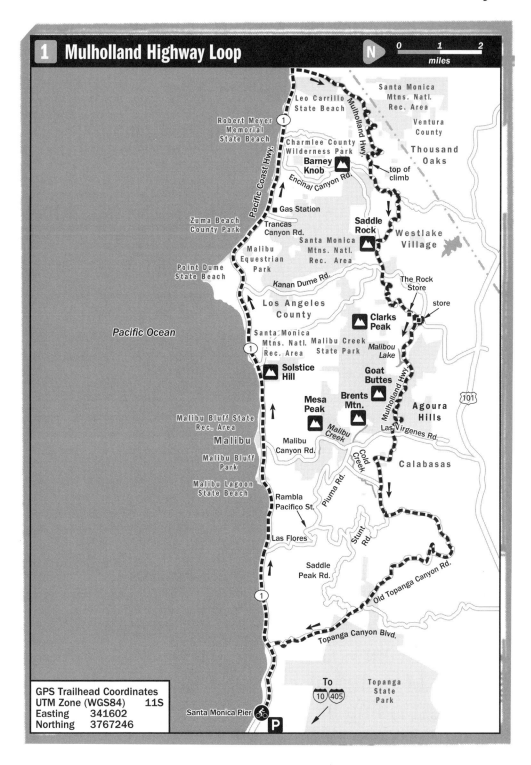

1 Mulholland Highway Loop

N

0   1   2
miles

Santa Monica
Mtns. Natl.
Rec. Area

Leo Carrillo
State Beach

Ventura
County

Robert Meyer
Memorial
State Beach

Charmlee County
Wilderness Park

Thousand
Oaks

**Barney
Knob**

top of
climb

Encinal Canyon Rd.

Pacific Coast Hwy.

Mulholland Hwy.

Gas Station

Zuma Beach
County Park

Trancas
Canyon Rd.

**Saddle
Rock**

Westlake
Village

Santa Monica
Mtns. Natl.
Rec. Area

Malibu
Equestrian
Park

Point Dume
State Beach

Kanan Dume Rd.

The Rock
Store

Los Angeles
County

store

**Clarks
Peak**

Pacific Ocean

Santa Monica
Mtns. Natl.
Rec. Area

Malibu Creek
State Park

Malibou
Lake

**Solstice
Hill**

**Goat
Buttes**

101

**Mesa
Peak**

**Brents
Mtn.**

Agoura
Hills

Las Virgenes Rd.

Malibu Bluff State
Rec. Area

Malibu

Malibu
Creek

Calabasas

Malibu Bluff
Park

Malibu
Canyon Rd.

Cold
Creek

Malibu Lagoon
State Beach

Piuma Rd.

Rambla
Pacifico St.

Las Flores

Stunt
Rd.

Saddle
Peak Rd.

Old Topanga Canyon Rd.

Topanga Canyon Blvd.

To

10 405

Topanga
State
Park

GPS Trailhead Coordinates
UTM Zone (WGS84)   **11S**
Easting   341602
Northing   3767246

Santa Monica Pier

P

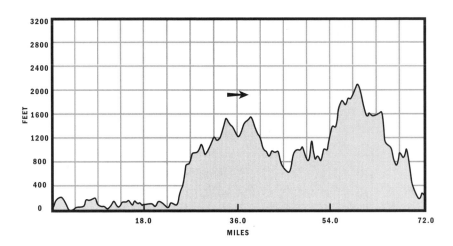

onto Pacific Coast Highway, or PCH. You may need to press the pedestrian-crossing button to get the light to change.

PCH has a wide shoulder almost every inch of the way up the coast into Ventura County. There will be one relatively narrow spot just north of Sunset Boulevard at Porto Marina Way, but otherwise you will enjoy a wide shoulder while riding north. Similarly, the road quality will be very good except—

These asphalt ribbons have it all: steep pitches, dramatic vistas, technical turns, and sweeping, no-brake descents. This is arguably some of the finest riding in the world.

once again—as you approach Porto Marina Way, where the surface is very rough and has some potholes.

PCH hugs the beach, at once giving you a gorgeous vantage of one of the world's great sections of coast and allowing you a mercifully flat ride—until you reach Malibu, whereupon a sharp hill rises up to Pepperdine University and Malibu Canyon Road. The hill averages roughly 8 percent for 0.4 miles. The next 2 miles roll up and down slightly until a downhill takes you back to sea level. At Corral Canyon Road, there is a gas station with all the necessities, though it is unlikely you will need to stop this early in the ride.

Continue west on PCH. You'll pass the turn onto Latigo Canyon Road, which is featured in another ride in this chapter. Following Latigo, you will encounter two gradually rolling hills followed by a steep descent to Zuma Beach that will have you traveling more than 35 mph. Another mile up on your right is a gas station, super-market, and coffee shop at Trancas Canyon Road. To the left is Broad Beach Road, which is the address of many a Hollywood star. To get on your way quickly, grab some water at the gas station. If you'd prefer to do some star sighting, get a latte at the coffee shop.

Another 5.5 miles up PCH you will encounter Leo Carillo State Beach and your turn onto the day's big attraction: Mulholland Highway. The climb up Mulholland is 7.3 miles and ascends 1,550 feet. That works out to an average gradient of only 4 percent, but thanks to a dip in the climb the riding is generally closer to 5 percent.

The twisting of the climb offers constantly changing views of Arroyo Sequit, including a few glimpses of the ocean. The lack of development makes the arroyo seem remote, so you may be surprised when you see a farm of enormous satellite dishes followed a little later by a golf course.

Upshift for a brief descent to an intersection where Mulholland Highway joins Decker Canyon Road briefly. Bear left at the intersection. The road will resume climbing almost immediately in a series of three rollers, gaining another 450 feet. Most of the time, this exposed section of road offers great views, but in the summer this canyon sheltered from the coastal air can heat up like the inside of a car on a July afternoon, reaching triple digits. Because the road isn't often flat, it is important to drink at every opportunity.

The road tops out 3.1 miles from the Decker-Mulholland intersection at just more than 2,000 feet of elevation. Yet another hill makes the next mile to the intersection with Encinal Canyon Road very tough. Mulholland intersects with Encinal. Turn left here, and although it will seem like you are turning onto Encinal, you will

be continuing on Mulholland. You will descend gently over the next mile before a short hill that rises to the intersection with Kanan Dume Road. Make good use of the opportunity to drink and eat.

After you cross Kanan Dume, you will encounter one final rise before you encounter one of the biggest descents of the day. After you gain less than 100 feet, Triunto Valley opens up before you. Less than a quarter-mile into the descent, there is a scenic pullout to your right that gives commanding views of the valley below.

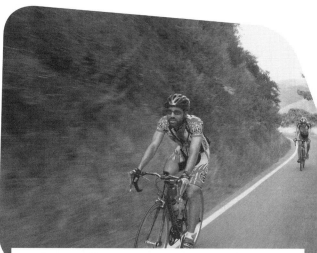

James Bedrosian and Jim Bowles enjoy a descent on Mulholland Highway.

It's worth the stop, especially if you are tired; you also get a view of the downhill to come. If you choose not to stop, try not to spin out your 12-tooth cog; the turns can't be taken at Formula 1 speeds. The descent on Mulholland into Triunto Valley slides 1,000 feet, with no fewer than eight switchbacks and numerous other bends and turns; the gradient is frequently 5 to 7 percent, but almost every one of the turns is banked. To say it's tricky is like saying a minefield isn't a great place for a hike.

After 2.5 miles of roller-coaster twists

and turns, the grade will ease and the turns end. Following a bit of runout, you will see Ed and Vern's Rock Store on your right. The Rock Store is an institution in Los Angeles motorcycle culture. While the gas pumps out front no longer work, no one seems to mind. People are there to show off their bikes (which range from Harleys to Ducattis) and to eat at the restaurant. It is known as a favorite hangout of *Tonight Show* host Jay Leno. Seemingly hewn from the rock of the canyon itself, the building and patio are something of a rustic wonder. You can get

Jim Bowles and James Bedrosian climb the long ascent of Mulholland Highway.

water here should you need it. However, you may want to pick up an energy drink or a snack; that opportunity is less than a mile up the road.

Turn left at Sierra Creek Road, which is straight and cruises slightly downhill to meet Kanan Dume Road. On the corner to your right is the Rustic Market, which is becoming popular with motorcyclists who think the Rock Store is too crowded. In addition to all the usual convenience-store offerings you'd expect, the market has a deli that will make a sandwich to order.

Go right out of the parking lot and take Kanan Dume a little more than 0.1 mile to Troutdale Road. Troutdale will take you

back to Mulholland in 0.3 miles, where you turn left to continue. Another 0.75 miles further on Mulholland is Lake Vista Drive. This 1.4-mile detour takes you by a stunning little neighborhood and Malibou Lake, which served as a film location for the movie *Must Love Dogs*. It's an idyllic hideaway worth seeing.

Turn right at Mulholland. The road will continue to wind through Triunto Canyon over two significant hills, the second of which will top out slightly more than 1,000 feet. A welcome respite follows with a lazily twisting descent to the intersection with Las Virgenes Road. Shift to your small chain ring before crossing Las Virgenes. The road will continue its constantly rolling texture. A few of these hills have the added interest of offering false crests before they gain even more height.

Your next turn is 4.3 miles from the intersection with Las Virgenes. Turn left onto Dry Canyon Cold Creek Road for the climb up what riders call "Seven-Minute Hill." Given that the climb gains more than 350 feet in only 2 miles (that's a less than 4 percent grade), most riders actually need more like 14 to 20 minutes. The name came from the professional riders of the old Mercury Team who used to train on these roads and would ascend Seven-Minute Hill in their big ring. Ouch.

Seven-Minute Hill rejoins Mulholland at a gated community (on the south side of Mulholland). There is a water spigot at the back of the guardhouse. Most of the guards will let you get water there if you ask. Mulholland straightens at this point for a steep descent (11 percent early on) to the right turn onto Dry Canyon Cold Creek Road. This turn is uphill and frequently sandy. Scrub your speed before heading into this turn.

While Dry Canyon Cold Creek is a very windy road (what's new?), it descends ever so slightly, again giving you a chance to eat and drink before tackling your final ascent of the day, Old Topanga. This climb will take you out of the canyon to begin your descent back to the coast. Old Topanga Canyon Road is a 1.5-mile climb and ascends a little more than 400 feet for an average gradient of 5 percent. The canyon is filled with a thick stand of oak trees, and if it is hot you will be grateful for the shade.

Following a sharp right turn at the top, there is an opportunity to pull off the road and recover from your effort, or you can just jump into the 4-mile descent to Topanga Canyon Road. The early part of the descent features the tightest turns. Following the third switchback, the descent becomes much easier, though it will be broken up by two short rises, both of which you should be able to take in your big ring.

At Topanga Canyon, turn right. There are two small markets 0.6 miles up the road: one on your right and another across on the left. With all the day's big challenges out of the way, you may not need to stop. The descent of Topanga Canyon is 3 miles, of which the first half is fairly steep. Even with a headwind blowing up the canyon, top speeds in excess of 40 mph are possible. However, the second half of the descent, while no less twisty, is considerably more flat; you can have some fun turning a big gear here. Be sure to stay to the right after the steep portion of the descent is over. Most cars won't attempt to pass you on the steep portion, but they will pass you once your speed drops.

Turn left at PCH. Surfers park on this side of the road, and you will find less room to negotiate than when you were riding northbound. Watch for surfboards and opening doors.

At Temescal Canyon, turn right into the parking lot of Will Rogers State Beach; there are openings for pedestrians to pass through the entry and exit lanes for cars. Ride up the ramp back onto the bike path. Your trip south to the parking will be short, and by this time the beach will be lively with other cyclists, skaters, surfers, and volleyball players.

After the Ride

From the pier's parking lot, you are a very short walk from a few restaurants to the south and several above you on the pier itself. For more selection and sightseeing, you can take the stairs up to the pier and then walk east to the Third Street Promenade. The promenade has a great array of restaurants, coffee shops, and ice cream parlors. Once your appetite is satisfied, you can take in the street performers and great clothing and book emporia.

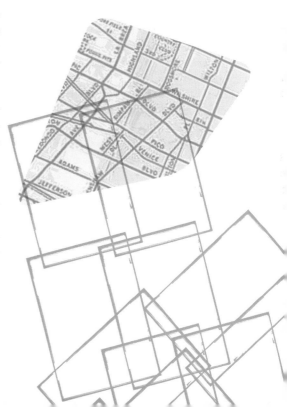

2 | Topanga Canyon Loop

AT A GLANCE

Length: 39 miles
Configuration: Loop
Difficulty: Difficult
Climbing: 3,700 feet

Maximum gradient: 12%

Scenery: Ocean, canyons, vineyards, and the Los Angeles coastline

Exposure: Usually sunny

Road traffic: Pacific Coast Highway is busy, but otherwise traffic is pretty light

Road surface: Generally good, though there can be occasional rockfall, resulting in some gravel near canyon walls

Riding time: 5 hours

Maps: Los Angeles County *Thomas Guide* pages 671, 631, 630, 590, 559, 589, and 629

In Brief

The Malibu coast is known for opulent homes owned by rich Hollywood stars. However, the community of Topanga is nestled in a canyon away from the coast. The area is rustic and alternative and carries an air of independence that harkens back to the hippie vibe of the 1960s. The canyon roads, which wind and twist through the mountains, are popular not only with cyclists but also with motorcycle and sports car enthusiasts. The climbs are difficult, and the descents challenging but thrilling.

Directions

This ride begins in Santa Monica at the world-famous Santa Monica Pier. Parking is inexpensive and plentiful, provided you arrive in the morning. To get to the pier, travel west on I-10 from I-405. Exit the 10 at Fourth Street and move into the left lane. Turn left at Colorado Avenue, proceed south two blocks, and turn right on Seaside Terrace. You will immediately see signs for parking. Free street parking isn't easy to find nearby.

Description

Ride north from the Santa Monica Pier parking lot and take the bike path that rings the lot. A number of beach homes and a bike-rental kiosk line the path, but then it bends left and traces a route away from commercial development. Continue north on this path to Will Rogers State Beach.

Here the bike path ends and you will head down a ramp and into the parking lot for the beach. There is a light at the parking lot entrance; you can press the crossing button at the left of the entrance to change it. Turn left out of the parking lot onto Pacific Coast Highway. Generally, the pavement here is good and the shoulder is wide, but for 0.3 miles after Sunset Boulevard, the pavement is very rough and there is one significant pothole.

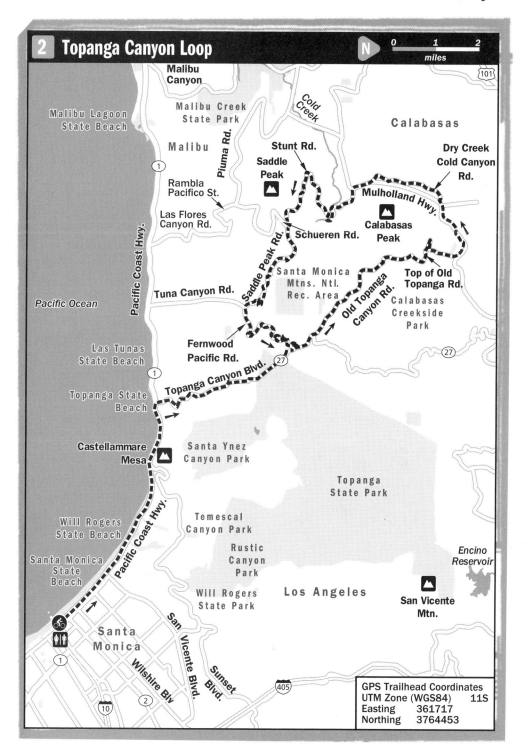

2 Topanga Canyon Loop

N

0   1   2
miles

Malibu Canyon

Cold Creek

Malibu Lagoon State Beach

Malibu Creek State Park

Calabasas

1

Piuma Rd.

Malibu

Stunt Rd.

Saddle Peak

Dry Creek Cold Canyon Rd.

Rambla Pacifico St.

Mulholland Hwy.

Las Flores Canyon Rd.

Schueren Rd.

Calabasas Peak

Pacific Coast Hwy.

Saddle Peak Rd.

Santa Monica Mtns. Ntl. Rec. Area

Top of Old Topanga Rd.

Tuna Canyon Rd.

Pacific Ocean

Old Topanga Canyon Rd.

Calabasas Creekside Park

Fernwood Pacific Rd.

27

27

Las Tunas State Beach

1

Topanga Canyon Blvd.

Topanga State Beach

Castellammare Mesa

Santa Ynez Canyon Park

Topanga State Park

Will Rogers State Beach

Temescal Canyon Park

Santa Monica State Beach

Pacific Coast Hwy.

Rustic Canyon Park

Encino Reservoir

Los Angeles

San Vicente Mtn.

Will Rogers State Park

San Vicente Blvd.

Santa Monica

1

Wilshire Blv

2

Sunset Blvd.

405

10

GPS Trailhead Coordinates	
UTM Zone (WGS84)	11S
Easting	361717
Northing	3764453

101

BICYCLING

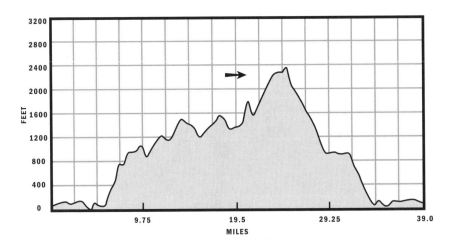

Approaching Topanga Canyon Boulevard, the road will rise and narrow. There are K-rails blocking some of the shoulder. This section of road seems to be perpetually under construction. Turn right onto Topanga Canyon Boulevard; there is a good, though narrow, shoulder. The road climbs gradually for the next 2.2 miles. Beware of expending too much energy on this false flat. Just after crossing Topanga Creek, the climb begins in earnest. For the next mile, you'll be climbing up a grade ranging between 8 and 12 percent. The worst is at the beginning, but, again, if you go too hard early, you'll suffer badly farther up.

In Topanga you will roll by two small markets at Fernwood Pacific Road. It's unlikely you'll need water this early, but it's good to know it's there. Half a mile beyond the markets is your next turn, left onto Old Topanga Canyon Road. This is another road that starts climbing gently. The false flat will seem interminable, but 1.2 miles into the climb, the road takes a sudden turn up. It's a short hill and is quickly followed by a downhill run into a right-hand

bend. The climbing resumes immediately, though. From the bottom of the hill to the top of the climb is 2.2 miles. You'll ascend a little more than 530 feet for an average gradient of 4.5 percent.

The shoulder gets a little wider at the top of the climb, and there's room to pull off and recover. The view to the east is largely blocked by rock. The road passes through a tiny notch, but once you roll out you'll see a sweeping view of the Calabasas Highlands. The descent isn't terribly technical, but the sixth turn down is a tight right switchback. You will need to slow more for this turn than for any of the others. As you continue on the descent, watch for a left turn onto Dry Canyon Cold Creek Road. The turn will come up before the descent has finished running out; be sure to watch for approaching traffic before executing your turn because you can't see very far up the road until you are right at the intersection.

Dry Canyon Cold Creek ascends slightly as it winds toward your next turn. On its right, it is bordered by the Viewpoint School, a very exclusive private school.

The road will become briefly steeper before dropping slightly to your next turn, left onto Mulholland Highway.

Mulholland has a shoulder here; because the road doesn't have many twists, what traffic does pass is likely to be going quite a bit faster than you. Immediately after your turn, the road will rise as a false flat; the grade will remain very gentle for more than 200 yards. But you knew that couldn't last. Following a right bend, the road will climb much more steeply, reaching a maximum grade of 11 percent, but fortunately the hill is mercifully short—less than 200 yards. At the top there is a gated community on the left. Behind the guardhouse is a water faucet; most of the guards will allow you to top off your bottles—if you ask first.

After having a drink and a bite to eat, cross Mulholland and pick up Dry Canyon Cold Creek once again. This is a fun little descent that takes you by some homes bound to make you question your career choice. A few of the turns are pretty tight, though banked. When Dry Canyon Cold Creek rejoins Mulholland, turn right. Ride 0.3 miles on Mulholland and then turn left on Stunt Road.

Stunt is a 4-mile climb that ascends more than 1,350 feet at an average gradient of 6 percent. There are two brief dips early in the climb, but following those there is no rest until you reach the intersection of Stunt Road, Saddle Peak Road, and Schueren Road. Charting your progress on a climb that can take a half-hour to ascend can be difficult. Fortunately, there are three painted markers on the surface of the road; the first comes when you are 3 km (1.8 miles) from the top. You will see two more 1 kilometer (0.6 miles) and 500 meters (0.3 miles) from the top of the climb.

Your sweeping view takes in Malibu Creek State Park. The park offers great hiking in a truly rural setting minutes from suburban Los Angeles. It was once owned

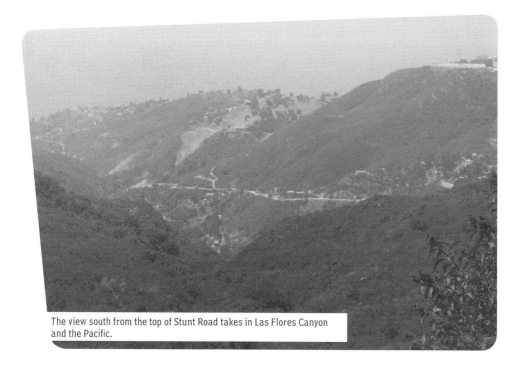

The view south from the top of Stunt Road takes in Las Flores Canyon and the Pacific.

by 20th Century Fox and used as a film location for a number of productions, including *Tora, Tora, Tora* and *Butch Cassidy and the Sundance Kid*. The television series *M*A*S*H** built its permanent set here.

At the top of Stunt, there is a broad parking area to the left of the intersection of the three roads. If you appreciate fine sports cars and motorcycles, you will enjoy the view at the top. This is a popular stopping point for drivers and riders of high-performance vehicles. Given the number of Ferraris and Ducattis that park here, one could be forgiven for thinking the Italian consulate was nearby.

There are two routes back to the coast; your route involves one more short climb before you slalom down to the coast. The exceptionally tired can avail themselves of another option and begin descending immediately by turning right on Schueren Road and then turning left on Rambla Pacifico Street. This descent is detailed further in the ride over Latigo and Piuma Canyons (ride 4, Latigo–Piuma Loop).

Roll out to your left onto Saddle Peak Road. The slope here varies between a false flat (with a grade of 1 to 3 percent) and utterly flat for the first few hundred yards. You will encounter a sharp right bend that begins the short (0.4-mile) climb to the top of Saddle Peak. The view here is among the best in all of Malibu because you're so close to Los Angeles. One can see not only the ocean and beaches but also the highlands of Pacific Palisades, Santa Monica, and even downtown.

Initially, the descent winds through several switchbacks. A mile down the descent you will round a left-sweeping turn and hit a slight rise. If you haven't scrubbed too much speed through braking, you will be able to make a short out-of-the-saddle effort to crest the rise and continue the descent.

Saddle Peak intersects with Tuna Canyon Road. Turn left and continue your descent— it is possible to turn right and descend Tuna Canyon to the coast, but this descent is very steep and technical, arguably the most difficult descent in Malibu . . . and that's saying

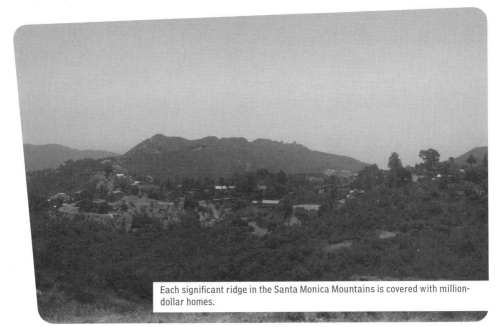

Each significant ridge in the Santa Monica Mountains is covered with million-dollar homes.

something. Following your left turn, you'll notice Tuna Canyon will become Fernwood Pacific Road. This 2.75-mile descent is very technical in its own right and contains 34 separate turns in that short span. The frequent turns through the enclave of Fernwood are complicated by the road's steep grade (7.4 percent, with pitches up to 14 percent) and the number of intersecting roads. Don't get too exuberant here; this is a fun descent, but even an experienced cyclist can get in over his head.

Fernwood Pacific Ts into Topanga Canyon Road. If you need water or food, there are two markets right here. This is also a safe spot to rest, out of the way, if your hands are tired from the previous descent. Turn right on Topanga Canyon. As you may recall from your earlier traverse of this road, it is flat for nearly a half-mile before your final descent commences. Traffic on Topanga Canyon is heavier than on any of the other canyon roads you have ridden on this loop. Once the descent begins in earnest, take the lane; cyclists' descending speeds can exceed 40 mph during the road's steepest section. Soon after, the grade will ease into a much gentler downhill.

At Pacific Coast Highway, turn left. If you left early in the day, you will notice a great deal more traffic now. Though there is a wide shoulder, much of the road back to Will Rogers Beach will be lined by surfers' parked cars. Keep an eye out for open doors and swinging surfboards. Despite the presence of surfers, cars, and boards, there is room enough on the shoulder to accommodate you safely.

At Temescal Canyon Road, turn right and enter the parking lot for Will Rogers Beach State Park. There is a break in the entrance lane to allow pedestrians and cyclists to enter the bike path. Ride up the short ramp and turn left for the short ride back to the Santa Monica Pier. By midday on the week-

ends, the beach is in full swing. You'll see some great volleyball being played, families out for bike rides with their kids, joggers, inline skaters, and of course surfers.

After the Ride
From the pier's parking lot, you are a very short walk from a few restaurants to the south and several above you on the pier itself. For more selection and sightseeing, you can take the stairs up to the pier and then walk east to the Third Street Promenade. The promenade has a great array of restaurants, coffee shops, and ice cream parlors. Once your appetite is satisfied, you can take in the street performers and also great clothing and book emporia.

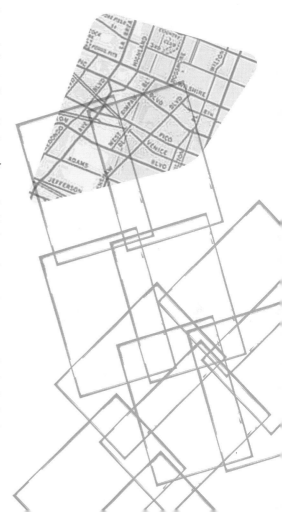

3 Point Mugu Out-and-Back

AT A GLANCE

Length: 44 miles

Configuration: Out-and-back

Difficulty: Moderate

Climbing: 1,700 feet

Maximum gradient: 9%

Scenery: Coastal vegetation, cactus, palm trees, beach, and ocean

Exposure: Extreme

Road traffic: Light to moderate

Road surface: Pretty good to excellent

Riding time: 3 hours

Maps: Los Angeles County *Thomas Guide* pages 671, 631, 630, 629, 628, 668, 667, 627, 626, 625 Ventura County *Thomas Guide* pages 387, and 584

In Brief

Pacific Coast Highway is certainly one of the world's great coastal roads. For 22 miles, the road rolls and weaves with the coastline. This stretch from Malibu to Point Mugu in Ventura County still holds the promise of an unspoiled California, a place where any dream might come true. It's a pilgrimage every roadie should make.

Directions

From the Westside: At the intersection of I-10 and I-405, travel west on the 10, going 4 miles, until it merges with Pacific Coast Highway. Drive north on PCH for 12.8 miles. At the top of a half-mile-long hill, turn left at Malibu Canyon Road and into Malibu Bluff State Park (also called Michael Landon Park). The park has free parking and bathrooms.

From the San Fernando Valley: At the intersection of I-405 and CA 101, drive north on the 101 (it will seem like you are driving west, mostly because you are), traveling 13.8 miles, and exit at Las Virgenes Road. Drive south on Las Virgenes 9.5 miles until Las Virgenes (which becomes Malibu Canyon) dead ends into Malibu Bluff State Park.

Description

Most of the rides in this guide really can't be recommended past midday for reasons that have to do entirely with self-preservation. This one is a rare exception. With the start point of the ride firmly in Malibu just at the point where traffic begins to thin, this ride can be enjoyed almost any time of day. That wouldn't be the case if this ride originated at the Santa Monica Pier, like other rides in this chapter. Should you wish to do this ride, but want to start from the pier, the same suggestion applies: start early to avoid the heavy traffic that develops on PCH. In addition to setting an early start, it's better to go on Saturday and Sunday than on weekdays.

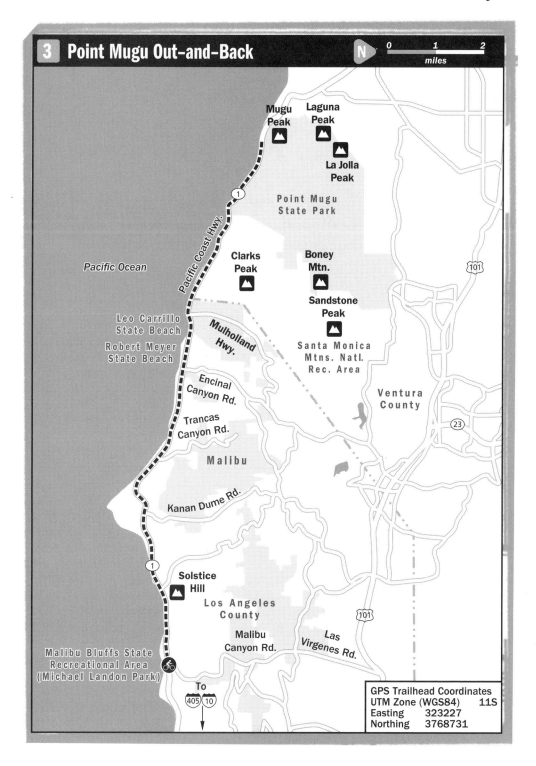

3 Point Mugu Out-and-Back

N

0   1   2
miles

Mugu Peak

Laguna Peak

La Jolla Peak

Point Mugu State Park

Pacific Ocean

Pacific Coast Hwy.

1

Clarks Peak

Boney Mtn.

101

Sandstone Peak

Leo Carrillo State Beach

Robert Meyer State Beach

Mulholland Hwy.

Santa Monica Mtns. Natl. Rec. Area

Ventura County

Encinal Canyon Rd.

Trancas Canyon Rd.

23

Malibu

Kanan Dume Rd.

1

Solstice Hill

Los Angeles County

Malibu Canyon Rd.

Las Virgenes Rd.

101

Malibu Bluffs State Recreational Area (Michael Landon Park)

To

405 10

GPS Trailhead Coordinates
UTM Zone (WGS84)   11S
Easting   323227
Northing   3768731

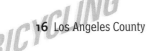
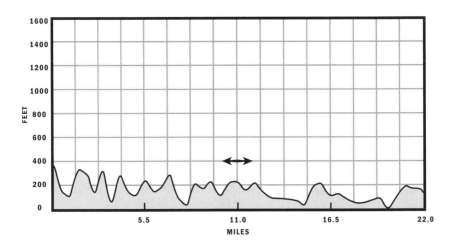

Out of Malibu Bluff State Park, turn left on PCH. You are at the top of a large bluff with a view of Pepperdine University sprawled on a beautifully manicured lawn opposite the park. One look at the surroundings and you'll understand that anyone who actually graduates from Pepperdine must truly be determined. PCH gently slopes downhill from here. The shoulder is wide, though it isn't very well tended. You'll see some potholes and cracks in the pavement, but even modest attention will keep you clear of trouble.

When dodging road hazards, keep in mind that traffic on PCH can travel at speeds ordinarily associated with some aircraft. While this isn't always the case, you should nevertheless always check over your shoulder before crossing into the traffic lane. Sad to say, some members of the local cycling community have been killed by careless drivers here.

Roughly 1.5 miles into the ride, PCH will begin a steep, right-bending descent. Check for traffic, and, provided conditions are clear, steer into the lane for the drop

to beach level. Most cyclists will spin out a 53 x 12, so taking the lane is an important part of staying safe because any debris on the shoulder will be difficult to dodge. Barely do you have time to enjoy the runout before the road begins its next hilly roll. Pass Latigo Canyon Road, which forms part of another great ride detailed in this chapter, on your right. At the intersection, the pavement bears the scar of spilled cement, which you will have to ride either over or around. In any case, do so cautiously.

Crest this next hill and shift back into your big chain ring for the next quick drop. Half a mile later, turn on the juice and use your momentum to carry you up the hill on the other side. This next hill lasts considerably longer; it's close to 3 miles. You are forgiven for wondering if the whole ride will be like this—it won't be. With 6 miles complete, you roll into another downhill, this one less severe than the last two. As you speed toward Zuma Beach, take the lane once again; there tends to be too much debris on the shoulder to be safe.

Another 1.5 miles along is a shopping

center on your right. Many cyclists who begin their ride in Santa Monica stop to get coffee here before turning around to head home. Those in need of a briefer stop usually choose the gas station at the light. After crossing Trancas Canyon Road, you'll find the landscape opens up some, with a bit of a field to the right. The road will continue to climb as a false flat for another 1.5 miles.

To your left, you can see a development of homes lining the beach. This is a very exclusive enclave of Malibu known as Broad Beach. Robert Redford, Dustin Hoffman, Walter Matthau, Whoopi Goldberg, and even Frank Sinatra have or have had homes here. The nearby coffee shop is a prime location to sight stars.

From the top of the rise past the gas station at the 9.5-mile mark you have another 4 miles of gently rolling terrain, and for a fair chunk you won't actually be able to see the coast. But suddenly you'll ease around a left bend and cruise down a half-mile run to Leo Carrillo Beach. As on almost all the other hills on this ride, the road immediately turns upward again to compensate for its loss in altitude. Depending on how ambitious you feel, this can be a fun hill to punch through in the big ring.

At around the 15-mile mark, you will cross the Ventura County line, and the coastline will come into view once again. At the intersection with Yerba Buena Road, there is a restaurant with some outdoor bathrooms that are usually open for cyclists to use. These will be the only facilities you will see for some miles to come.

This section of road leading to Point Mugu is what this ride is all about. The asphalt is in pristine shape, the shoulder unfurls to either side like a king-size sheet, and the combination of cliffs to your right and coastline just

yards from the edge of the road makes for an impossibly gorgeous ride. Although the road will continue to rise and drop on its serpentine course to Point Mugu, the change in elevation is absolutely minimal; wind is likely to be a much bigger influence. Those who start early are likely to enjoy minimal wind on the way out and benefit from a tailwind on the way back.

In the final 3 miles that lead to Point Mugu, the road is so nice and the bends so enjoyable that it's easy to want to hit the jets and hammer the distance to the rock. Don't make that mistake. Throttle back and enjoy the view. This is a section you really can't ride too slowly. Breathe in the scent of sea spray and look out along the ridgeline of the last of the Santa Monica Mountains as they lead to the Pacific.

PCH passes through a notch between Point Mugu, "the rock," and the mountains to the right. When safe, turn left into the parking area. There are no facilities here, but it's a "must stop" simply for the view. Have a bite, take a look around, and then head for the shoulder. Getting home is as easy as it gets: turn around. You have executed the second of the ride's three turns.

The big news about the ride back is that, with two exceptions, every hill you

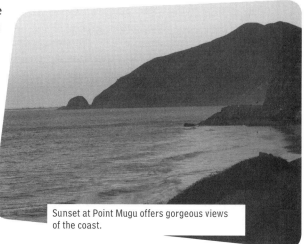

Sunset at Point Mugu offers gorgeous views of the coast.

descended on the way out is gentler than the hill you climbed. At the 30-mile mark you return to Leo Carrillo State Beach; as you climb away from the beach, dig a bit just so you won't bog down in the big ring. The easterly winds that blow the waves out in Santa Monica, Venice, and Manhattan Beach parallel the coast in Malibu. For cyclists, this means that, as the inland warms and the winds pick up, what begins as a light breeze becomes a full-blown tailwind. You'll gain a full cog on many hills on your way back. The later in the day you leave, the more pronounced this effect is.

Passing Zuma Beach, you encounter what was a fun descent on the way out. As a climb, it's a little tougher. The mile goes quickly and is made more pleasant by a wide shoulder. Those wanting a great view of the coast should turn right on Westward Beach Road. Turn left at Birdview Drive for a steep 0.3-mile climb up to the top of the cliffs. Birdview turns left a half-mile along and becomes the aptly named Cliffside Drive; slow down and drink in the spectacular views of the coast. Turn left on Fernhill Drive and left again Wildlife Road. Wildlife will T into Zumirez Drive (Barbara Streisand's compound is at the other end of this road). Bear left onto Zumirez and turn right immediately onto PCH.

The detour rejoins the main route past the top of the hill, so either path is a descent. It's a big relief. Following a brief flat, the road drops again, this time rather steeply, and immediately turns back up. Keep an eye out for cars entering from the right. There's a restaurant that serves a popular brunch here, and there's always a chance that a diner had one too many mimosas. Cresting the hill is a humbling event, involving successive downshifts before you finally concede the little ring.

Your final downhill opens up to beach to your right. Enjoy the final mile of easy pedaling before tackling the hill back up to the park. It's not a long climb, but the 175 feet of elevation gain forces almost everyone into a tiny gear.

After the Ride

Malibu has quite a selection of open-air restaurants. There are two primary commercial developments nearby. One is at Webb Way, south of PCH and barely a mile away, and the other is north of PCH at Cross Creek Road. Enjoy a meal and maybe follow it up with a walk on the beach.

This stretch from Malibu to Point Mugu in Ventura County still holds the promise of an unspoiled California, a place where any dream might come true.

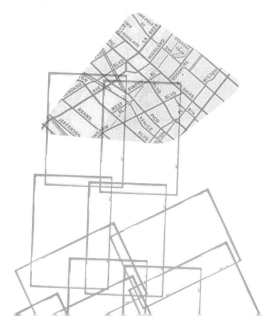

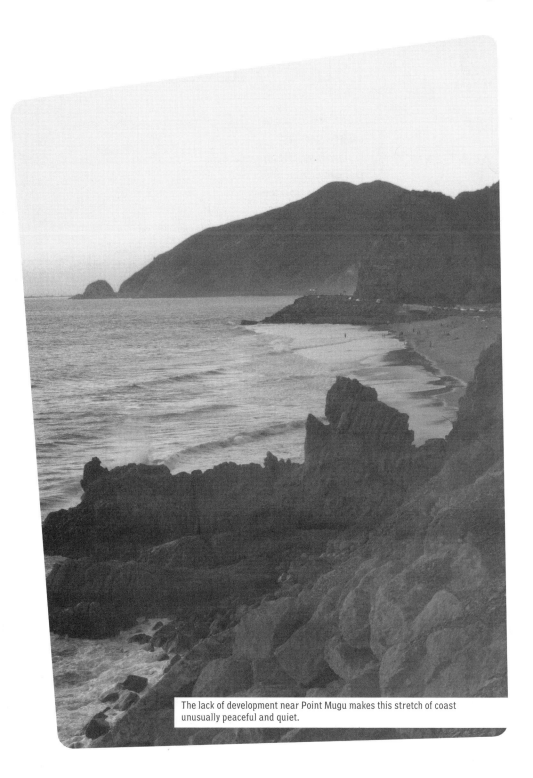

The lack of development near Point Mugu makes this stretch of coast unusually peaceful and quiet.

4 Latigo–Piuma Loop

AT A GLANCE

Length: 57 miles

Configuration: Loop

Difficulty: Difficult

Climbing: 4,600 feet

Maximum gradient: 12%

Scenery: Ocean, canyons, vineyards, and the Los Angeles coastline

Exposure: Usually sunny

Road traffic: Pacific Coast Highway is busy, but otherwise traffic is pretty light

Road surface: Generally good, though there can be occasional rockfall resulting in some gravel near canyon walls

Riding time: 4 hours

Maps: Los Angeles County *Thomas Guide* pages 671, 631, 630, 629, 628, 627, 587, and 588

In Brief

The canyon roads of Malibu haven't got the reputation of its surf, but they ought to. These asphalt ribbons have it all: steep pitches, dramatic vistas, technical turns, and sweeping, no-brake descents. This is arguably some of the finest riding in the world. These two canyon roads are popular not only with cyclists but also with motorcyclists and sports car enthusiasts. The two climbs will take you above 2,000 feet, making this one of the tougher routes in this book. That said, this ride is worth every drop of sweat you'll surrender; the views are truly world class.

Directions

This ride begins in Santa Monica at the world-famous Santa Monica Pier. Parking is inexpensive and plentiful, provided you arrive in the morning. To get to the pier, travel west on I-10 from I-405. Take the Fourth Street exit and move into the left lane. Turn left on Colorado Avenue, proceed south two blocks, and turn right on Seaside Terrace. You will immediately see signs for parking. Free street parking is hard to find around here.

Description

Like many rides in this book, this loop is easier and safer if you ride it in the morning because you'll ride the outbound leg against the morning traffic flow—into Los Angeles—and it will be cooler. Weekend mornings are preferable to weekday mornings, though the latter can be good if you start the ride after rush hour, which ends by around 9 a.m.

The ride begins on the beach bike path, which skirts the parking lot on its west and north sides. Ride 2.9 miles north (the ocean will be to your left) on the bike path. When you reach the parking lot at Temescal Canyon Road, exit the bike path and turn left onto Pacific Coast Highway. You may

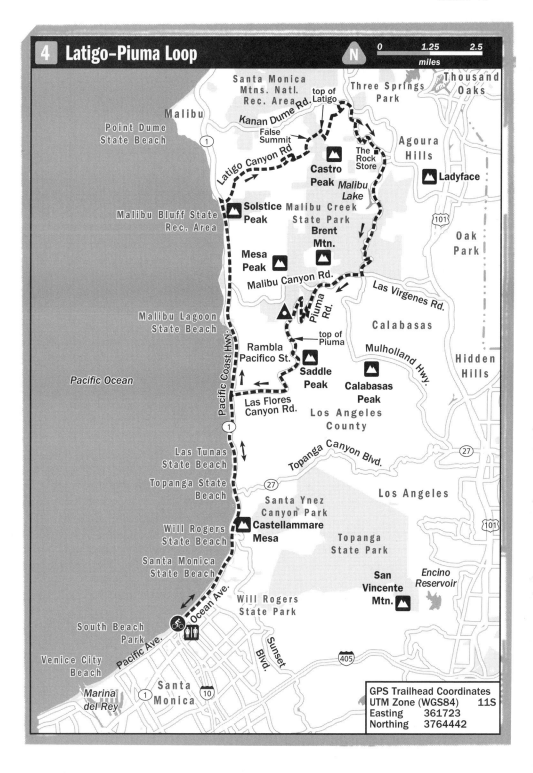

4 **Latigo–Piuma Loop**

N

0   1.25   2.5
miles

Santa Monica
Mtns. Natl.
Rec. Area
top of
Latigo

Three Springs
Park

Thousand
Oaks

Malibu

Point Dume
State Beach

Kanan Dume Rd.

False
Summit

Agoura
Hills

Latigo Canyon Rd.

The
Rock
Store

Castro
Peak

Malibu
Lake

Ladyface

Malibu Bluff State
Rec. Area

Solstice
Peak

Malibu Creek
State Park

Brent
Mtn.

101

Oak
Park

Mesa
Peak

Malibu Canyon Rd.

Malibu Lagoon
State Beach

Piuma Rd.

Las Virgenes Rd.

Calabasas

top of
Piuma

Pacific Ocean

Pacific Coast Hwy.

Rambla
Pacifico St.

Saddle
Peak

Mulholland Hwy.

Calabasas
Peak

Hidden
Hills

Las Flores
Canyon Rd.

Los Angeles
County

Las Tunas
State Beach

Topanga Canyon Blvd.

27

Topanga State
Beach

27

Los Angeles

Will Rogers
State Beach

Santa Ynez
Canyon Park

Castellammare
Mesa

Topanga
State Park

101

Santa Monica
State Beach

San
Vincente
Mtn.

Encino
Reservoir

South Beach
Park

Ocean Ave.

Will Rogers
State Park

Venice City
Beach

Pacific Ave.

Sunset Blvd.

405

Marina
del Rey

1

Santa
Monica

10

GPS Trailhead Coordinates
UTM Zone (WGS84)   11S
Easting   361723
Northing   3764442

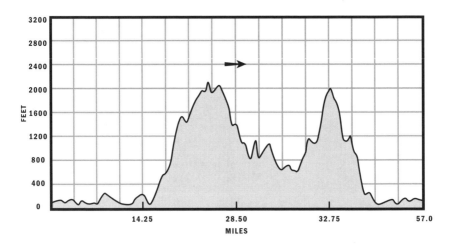

have to press the pedestrian crossing button to switch the light here.

PCH has a wide shoulder almost every inch of the way up the coast into Ventura County. There will be one relatively narrow spot just north of Sunset Boulevard at Porto Marina Way, but, otherwise, you will enjoy a wide shoulder while riding north. Similarly, the road quality will be very good except—once again—as you approach Porto Marina Way, where the surface is very rough and has some potholes.

PCH hugs the beach, at once giving you a gorgeous view of one of the world's great coastlines and allowing you a mercifully flat ride. That is, flat until you reach Malibu, whereupon a sharp hill rises up to Pepperdine University and Las Virgenes Road. The hill averages roughly 8 percent for 0.4 miles. The next 2 miles roll slightly until a downhill that takes you back to sea level. At Corral Canyon Road, there is a gas station with all the necessities, though it is unlikely you will need to stop this early in the ride. That said, you won't find water or a civilized bathroom again until you reach the Rock Store on Mulholland, some 14 miles away.

Roughly 0.7 miles from the gas station is the right turn that begins the climb up Latigo Canyon. The climb up Latigo is the longest in the Santa Monica Mountains, measuring 9.25 miles from its base and ascending 2,000 vertical feet. For the most part, the climb is gentle, averaging only 4.6 percent, but it has pitches as steep as 12 percent. It is one of the few climbs that offer the overexuberant an opportunity to recover from an effort and then make another big push. Perhaps the climb's best feature is that the road constantly turns and bends around the canyon, offering ever-changing views of the canyon itself and the coast below. If one thing about this climb is certain, it is that the road is anything but boring.

The first significant feature of the climb is a slight downhill that comes 5 miles in. While it doesn't last long—maybe a minute—it's just enough to let the legs recover some; you'll feel much better going into the next pitch. Soon after, you will see one of several vineyards visible on the ride. The Santa Monica Mountains aren't thought of as prime wine-growing territory, but some areas are, in fact, capable of producing enjoyable wines. This particular vineyard is devoted to cabernet sauvignon, merlot, and cabernet franc.

At 6.8 miles you crest a false summit; the way the road turns flat so suddenly, it is easy to think the climb is over. However, there is a short descent that follows, and then a final 1.2-mile push to the top. Be careful on the descent. There are three significant right-hand bends; the second and third feature decreasing-radius turns that can catch a rider off guard, and a fistful of rear brake has sent many riders to the ground.

The long, gentle grades of Latigo Canyon make climbing in a group possible and more enjoyable.

Following a sweeping left-hand switch-back that signals the end of the respite, the road dramatically ascends, and tight bends hide the pass from your view until nearly the last possible moment. The pass is on a right-hand bend; if you choose to stop, pull off the road fully to avoid being hit by passing cars whose drivers can tend toward the impatient.

The descent of Latigo to Kanan Dume Road is short—only 3 miles—but it is quick and technical. About two thirds of the way down, there is a sharp left-hand switchback followed by a sharp right-hand turn: watch

out for those. And when you see the sign for the stop ahead, immediately begin braking; you don't want to overshoot the stop and run into the road. Turn right on Kanan Dume and ride the half-mile (which includes one short roller) to Mulholland Highway and turn right again.

The nature of these canyon roads makes this area rather remote relative to the sprawling metropolis of Los Angeles. Don't make the mistake of running the stop signs or lights out here. The area is regularly patrolled by police on the lookout for speeding motorcycles and sports cars. Running any of the lights or stop signs can be both expensive and perilous.

Mulholland Highway is rarely flat; it undulates constantly and at times gains (or loses) hundreds of feet of elevation on a single hill. In addition to that, you'll find that the road bends and twists with the geography of the canyon. With a ridgeline separating this land from the ocean, the foliage reflects the desert climate of the region. You'll see sage and piñon and also many oak trees. You'll also run across many species of cactus. For most of the year, any grass you see is likely to be brown, unless, of course, it is part of someone's well-manicured yard. Accordingly, with a line of mountains separating the atmosphere of this valley from the ocean air, temperatures will be noticeably higher during the warm months, often averaging 10°F higher than at the beach. This difference can be even greater on especially hot days, or in the winter. The valley can lock in the cold air, yielding some surprises for those who aren't prepared.

Roughly 2.7 miles along Mulholland, you will reach The Rock Store. This is a restaurant that is an institution among area motorcyclists. For cyclists, it is an opportunity to find a bathroom and some water plus spy the latest in carbon-fiber motorcycle technology. From vintage Harleys to the newest Ducattis, you'll see it all here.

This stretch of Mulholland is 9 miles long and, because of the rollers, it is easy to push too hard up a hill, only to discover yet another around the next bend. Ride conservatively here so that you have something in reserve for the Piuma climb. At Las Virgenes Road, turn right; you'll have just more than a mile to the left turn onto Piuma Road.

Piuma quickly turns uphill. However, if you need water you have an opportunity to get some at a fountain in front of the Monte Nido fire station at the intersection with Cold Canyon Road. Have a seat on the bench and enjoy a bottle and some food before tackling the climb up Piuma. This climb isn't as long as Latigo, but at 5.2 miles, it is a lengthy ascent. And because it averages 6 percent with no flat spots to allow real recovery, your effort will be constant.

The road will constantly turn and twist during the climb, but what will be most helpful to you in charting your progress is tracking the four distinct switchbacks. Also, markers have been painted on the road counting down the final kilometers of the climb; you'll see white signs giving the 4k, 2k, 1k, 500m, 200m, and 100m markers. As you approach the fourth and final switchback, your view will be of the mountains of Malibu Creek State Park to the west. If the scene looks oddly familiar, there's a reason: if you were a viewer of the TV show M*A*S*H*, you saw these mountains at the start of each episode.

Upon exiting the fourth switchback, you will be at 1,300 feet, with 900 feet yet to ascend. Views here are much more exposed; you can look to your left and see the San Fernando Valley, and to your right your first opportunities to view Malibu Canyon's path to the coast emerge. There are a few opportunities to pull off on the right shoulder for dramatic views of

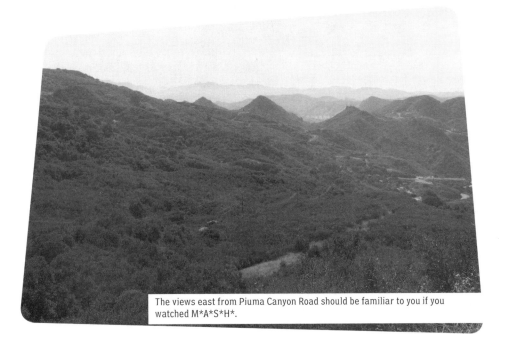

The views east from Piuma Canyon Road should be familiar to you if you watched M*A*S*H*.

... this ride is worth every drop of sweat you'll surrender; the views are truly world class.

the beach below; they are worth slowing down for, if not for stopping.

When riding the knife-ridge edge of the mountains, you can encounter some unusual climatic conditions because cool air coming off the ocean pushes up against the Santa Monica Mountains as the sun heats the air in the San Fernando Valley. When that air is hot enough, it will draw the cool, moist air off the ocean and over the ridge, causing a fogbank.

The top of Piuma is entirely exposed and doesn't offer particularly good views of the coast. On the left there is a gated development, and there is enough shoulder to pull off and have a drink and a bite to eat while you view the road below—the road you just conquered.

When you resume your path on Piuma, the road serpentines seaward. Initially, the descent isn't difficult, but that changes when you reach Las Flores Canyon Road, 1.6 miles into the drop. The 4-mile descent of Las Flores averages more than 8 percent, but that's not the big news: there are sections of this descent as steep as 18 percent. Be sure to brake before initiating turns, and watch for rockfall on the road. When you reach PCH, use the crossing button to change the light, otherwise you'll be standing there for quite some time.

The shoulder on PCH southbound isn't as wide as on the northbound side, and, worse still, this side is where the majority of

surfers park. Watch for opening doors, as lots of people will be stowing and removing surfboards from vehicles. Fortunately, you should get through this section relatively quickly; most days there's a prevailing tailwind.

At Temescal Canyon, turn right into the parking lot; you'll notice openings for pedestrians to pass through the entry and exit lanes for cars. Pass through these crosswalks and ride up the ramp back onto the bike path. Your trip south to the parking lot will be short, and by this time the beach will be lively with other cyclists, skaters, surfers, and volleyball players; it's as vibrant a stretch of beach as you will find.

After the Ride

From the Santa Monica Pier's parking lot, you are a very short walk from a few restaurants to the south and several above you on the pier itself. For more selection and sightseeing, you can take the stairs up to the pier and then walk east to the Third Street Promenade. The promenade has a wide array of restaurants, coffee shops, and ice cream parlors. Once your appetite is satisfied, you can take in the street performers and the great clothing and book emporia.

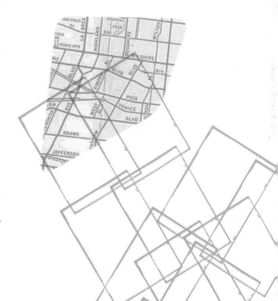

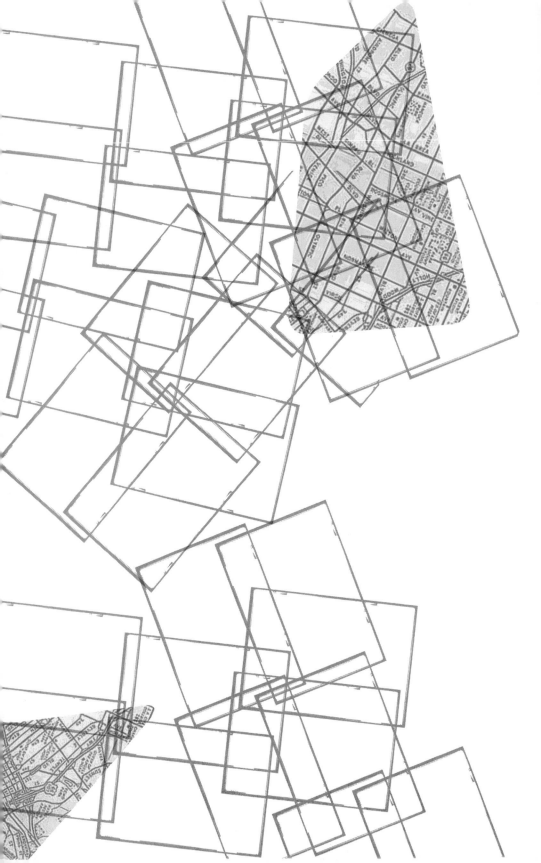

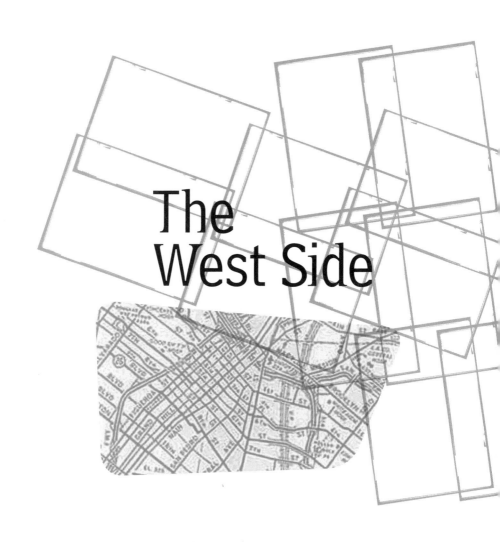

The
West Side

5

Ballona Creek Bike Path

AT A GLANCE	**Length:** 6 miles
	Configuration: One-way
	Difficulty: Easy
	Climbing: Less than 100 feet

Maximum gradient: 6%

Scenery: The wetlands of Ballona Creek, waterfowl, and the geometric concrete forms of Ballona Creek

Exposure: Mornings and late afternoons can be overcast

Road traffic: None

Road surface: Excellent

Riding time: 30 minutes

Maps: Los Angeles County *Thomas Guide* pages 702, 672, and 632

In Brief

The Ballona Creek Bike Path is a shortish bike path that, like many bike paths in Los Angeles County, parallels a waterway. In this case, the waterway is Ballona Creek, which empties into the Pacific at Marina Del Rey. It is an excellent way to ride inland from the coast for those headed to Westside destinations and is popular with riders from Beverly Hills heading south to the Baldwin Hills.

Directions

Take I-405 north to CA 90 west. Exit at Culver Boulevard. Turn left and take Culver southwest 2 miles to Vista Del Mar. It will appear that Culver bears left at the light; that is, in fact, Vista Del Mar. Bear slightly right to continue on Culver. Turn right on Pacific Avenue and begin looking for street parking. Pacific Avenue dead-ends at the bridge.

Description

This bike path tracks a northeast route from Marina Del Rey into Culver City. From a bike-commuting standpoint, it is very useful and offers riders relatively easy access to and from many Westside destinations, including Century City, Beverly Hills, and all points in Culver City.

Unfortunately, Culver City isn't always the safest place on the planet. If you plan to ride this path very far inland, it is a good idea to have a friend along; riders have reported fewer problems closer to the beach. This is definitely not a bike path to ride after nightfall.

From a scenic standpoint, the path's greatest points of interest are along the first 1.4 miles extending from the coast, where the course hugs the southern edge of the Ballona Creek Wetlands. This hotly contested preserve has been ground zero for some contentious fights between (big surprise) real estate developers and (who

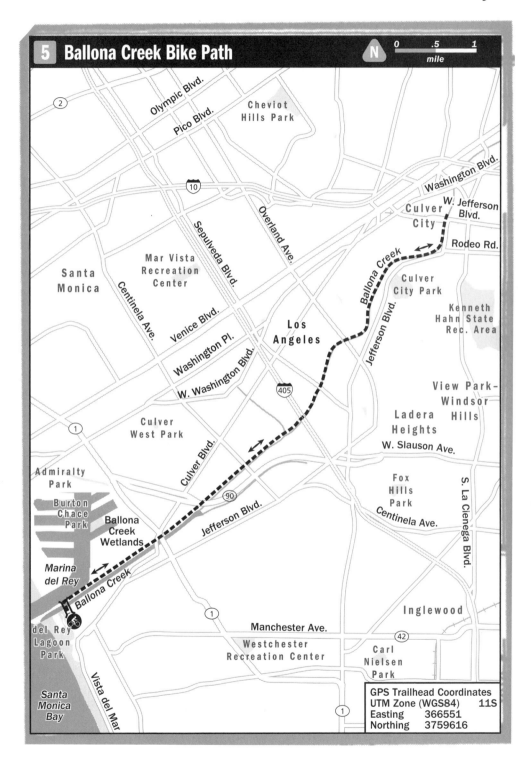

5 **Ballona Creek Bike Path**

N

0   .5   1
mile

Olympic Blvd.

Pico Blvd.

Cheviot
Hills Park

Washington Blvd.

10

W. Jefferson
Blvd.

Culver
City

Rodeo Rd.

Overland Ave.

Sepulveda Blvd.

Ballona Creek

Mar Vista
Recreation
Center

Culver
City Park

Kenneth
Hahn State
Rec. Area

Santa
Monica

Centinela Ave.

Venice Blvd.

Los
Angeles

Jefferson Blvd.

Washington Pl.

W. Washington Blvd.

405

View Park–
Windsor
Hills

Ladera
Heights

1

Culver
West Park

Culver Blvd.

W. Slauson Ave.

Admiralty
Park

90

Fox
Hills
Park

Centinela Ave.

S. La Cienega Blvd.

Burton
Chace
Park

Ballona
Creek
Wetlands

Jefferson Blvd.

Marina
del Rey

Ballona Creek

del Rey
Lagoon
Park

1

Inglewood

Manchester Ave.

42

Santa
Monica
Bay

Vista del Mar

Westchester
Recreation Center

Carl
Nielsen
Park

1

GPS Trailhead Coordinates
UTM Zone (WGS84)   11S
Easting   366551
Northing   3759616

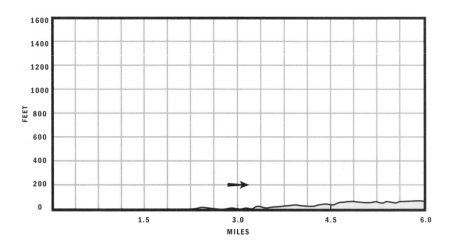

else?) conservationists. The argument that the coastal estuary is so tiny (the wetlands are only 186 acres of what was once more than 2,100 acres) that it can't support any significant wildlife seems rational. After all, the expanse of Los Angeles is beating at its door—that is, until you actually spend a few minutes looking through the fence at the idyllic treasure. Currently, private foundations are working to restore the reserve to 340 acres.

Some of the most common flora include willows, bulrush, Fremont cottonwood, cattails, and tule. Coastal sage scrub is a

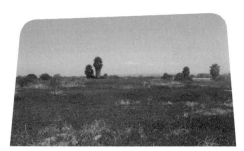

The Ballona Wetlands are an unusual oasis within urban Los Angeles.

component of the environment and includes a more unusual collection of plants, such as coastal prickly pear cactus, bush lupine, deerweed, laurel sumac, and coyote brush.

The restoration project is receiving cooperation from a number of state agencies. Nonnative species (both plants and predators) are being removed with the hope that species that once proliferated will return. California least tern once nested there but no longer do. Conservationists hope that replanting cord grass and other native species will attract the birds, along with the El Segundo blue butterfly and the Southwestern willow flycatcher. However, no one visits a wetland for the species that may return.

The area boasts 215 different species of bird. Commonly seen types include mallard ducks, red-tailed hawks, kingfishers, ring-billed gulls, and rock and mourning doves. With a little patience, you can see a few different varieties of hummingbirds, swallows, warblers, flycatchers, finches, and sparrows, and a huge assortment of shore birds.

Most of the mammals in the ecosystem are small; rabbits and mice proliferate. However, fox, skunk, and raccoon have been sighted.

The bike path edges the preserve for what seems entirely too short a stretch and borders Ballona Creek to its south. Unfortunately, the creek itself looks more like an Army Corps of Engineers project than it does a living waterway. The concrete spillway may have something to do with that. When the water is low (which is most of the time) the creek becomes nothing more than an expanse of white concrete.

The north side of the bike path passes behind a series of businesses in Culver City before commercial development gives way to residential development and schools. The path has 11 distinct exits along its course, including the final one at Jefferson Boulevard. Note that there is usually a bar

or a short section of chain-link fence that forces the rider to dismount and carry the bicycle over the barrier. It may be a bit annoying, but it does keep motorcycle traffic off the path.

Like other bike paths, this path crosses major thoroughfares via underpasses that add a bit of pedaling interest to what would otherwise be a very flat route. Afternoon rides have the added dimension of an offshore wind. Anyone riding toward the coast in the afternoon will notice a stiff headwind.

The northeast terminus of the bike path is at Jefferson Boulevard. From a navigational point of view, the location is very convenient. Jefferson intersects La Cienega, Venice, and Washington boulevards nearby. However, without a specific destination in mind and a preplanned route, this is no time to go explore. This is a more urban part of town with heavy traffic.

After the Ride

At the coastal end of the bike path, a right turn will deliver you to Fiji Way and Fisherman's Village, a touristy little development with some shops and a selection of restaurants. Riding straight on the jetty and crossing the bridge will take you to the restaurants that line Culver Boulevard near its intersection with Vista Del Mar just a few hundred yards from where you parked.

Fisherman's Village is a pleasant place to stop for a snack while riding on the West Side.

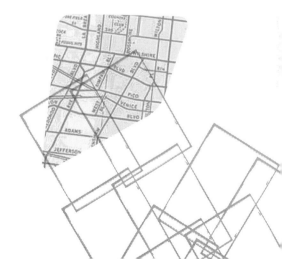

6

Santa Monica Beach Bike Path

AT A GLANCE

Length: 9.5 miles (one way)

Configuration: Out-and-back

Difficulty: Easy

Climbing: 150 feet

Maximum gradient: 3%

Scenery: Beach, ocean, an enormous marina full of boats, and the crowd at Venice Beach

Exposure: Mornings can be overcast

Road traffic: Very light

Road surface: Good, except for the asphalt in Marina Del Rey

Riding time: 40 minutes

Maps: Los Angeles County *Thomas Guide* pages 671, 631, and 630

In Brief

The Santa Monica Beach Bike Path extends from Will Rogers State Beach, at its northern terminus, south through Venice and Marina Del Rey to the bridge that crosses Ballona Creek. Along the way, you can see professional and aspiring volleyball players competing, body builders lifting at Muscle Beach, drum circles in Venice, sunbathers galore, and, if you're out early enough, the crew teams from University of California, Los Angeles and University of Southern California out rowing on Ballona Creek.

Directions

This ride begins in Santa Monica at the world-famous Santa Monica Pier. Parking is inexpensive and plentiful, provided you arrive in the morning. To get to the pier from points north and east: Travel west on I-10 from I-405. Exit I-10 at Fourth Street and move into the left lane. Turn left at Colorado Avenue and proceed south two blocks, then turn right on Seaside Terrace. You will immediately see signs for parking. Free street parking is hard to find nearby.

Parking is also available farther north on Pacific Coast Highway (PCH) at Will Rogers State Beach, which is reachable by continuing west on I-10 until it becomes PCH. Travel 2 miles north and turn left into the beach parking lot at Temescal Canyon. Parking is also available at the southern end of the bike path near the bridge, in Playa Del Rey.

From points south: Take I-405 north, to CA 90 west. Exit at Culver Boulevard. Turn left and take Culver southwest 2 miles to Vista Del Mar. It will appear that Culver bears left at the light; that is, in fact, Vista Del Mar. Bear slightly right to continue on Culver. Turn right on Pacific Avenue and begin looking for street parking. Pacific Avenue dead-ends at the bridge.

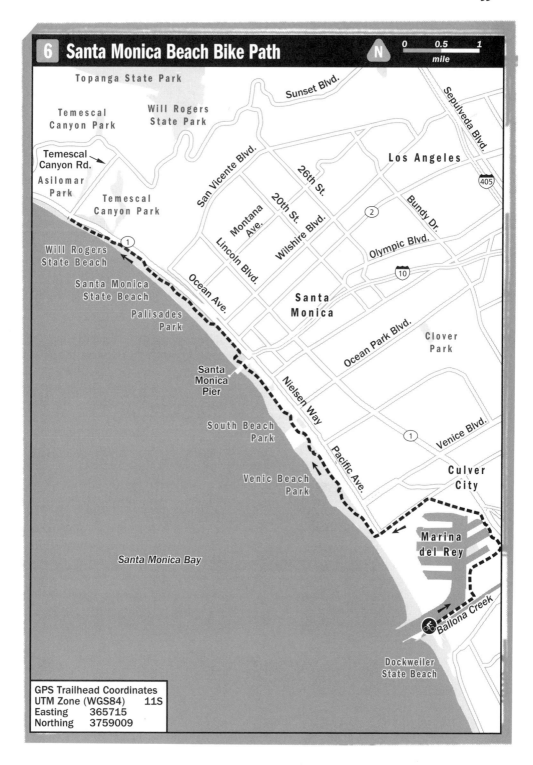

6 Santa Monica Beach Bike Path

N

0   0.5   1
mile

Topanga State Park

Sunset Blvd.

Sepulveda Blvd.

Temescal
Canyon Park

Will Rogers
State Park

Los Angeles

Temescal
Canyon Rd.

San Vicente Blvd.

26th St.

405

Asilomar
Park

Bundy Dr.

Temescal
Canyon Park

20th St.

2

Montana
Ave.

Wilshire Blvd.

Olympic Blvd.

1

Will Rogers
State Beach

Lincoln Blvd.

10

Santa Monica
State Beach

Ocean Ave.

Santa
Monica

Palisades
Park

Clover
Park

Ocean Park Blvd.

Santa
Monica
Pier

Nielsen Way

South Beach
Park

Pacific Ave.

1

Venice Blvd.

Venic Beach
Park

Culver
City

Marina
del Rey

Santa Monica Bay

Ballona Creek

Dockweiler
State Beach

GPS Trailhead Coordinates
UTM Zone (WGS84)   11S
Easting   365715
Northing   3759009

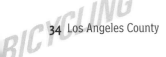

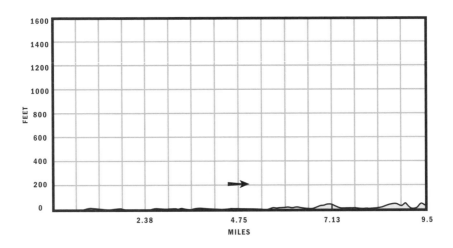

Bike Rental

Visitors to Los Angeles can rent bicycles at six locations along the path. There is one just north of the Santa Monica Pier along the path, and there is another just south of the pier along the walkway that passes under the pier.

Description

This ride has the distinction of being both the flattest ride in this guide (there is less than 150 feet of elevation gain from one end to the other) and the most endlessly entertaining. If you like to people watch, this stretch of bike path could take most of the day to ride out and back. This description will take you through the route from the bridge in Marina Del Rey to its northern terminus at Will Rogers State Beach. You can ride any portion of the route with little fear of getting lost; it has few turns. And restroom facilities are plentiful along the path; you will never be more than a few hundred yards from one.

The Ballona Creek Bridge joins the South Bay Bike Path to the Santa Monica Beach Bike Path. In the early morning, the bridge is a great place to watch the crew teams rowing up and down Ballona Creek. At the northern end of the bridge is a jetty that separates Ballona Creek from the Marina Del Rey channel. You can see boats entering and leaving the marina along this stretch; some of them are truly impressive yachts. Looking to the northeast, you will get your first views of the marina itself.

Less than a mile into your ride, you'll notice the bike path bend to the left and can see it is possible to continue riding east. Bear left. The eastern continuation of the path is the Ballona Creek Bike Path, which, although popular with bicycle commuters and local residents who wish to ride on the beach bike path, isn't particularly scenic.

The bike path will end at Fiji Way. Exit the path and bear right onto Fiji. You will pass Fisherman's Village, a quaint collection of shops and restaurants with architecture that evokes the feel of an old wharf, on your left. Fiji Way will bend to the right, and approximately a half-mile up you will see markings on the road for the bike path, indicating a left turn. Fiji is very lightly traveled, and you should have no problem getting into the left-turn lane and turning up the ramp to the bike path's continuation. The asphalt here has some bumps and breaks, but because it hugs basins F, G, and H of Marina Del Rey, it is a fun and intimate view of the boating community. The path will cross Mindanao Way and Bali Way. Be sure to stop before crossing the streets.

After crossing Bali Way, the path will approach the Marina Del Rey library and cross Admiralty Way. There is a crossing signal here; you'll find the button on the right. The next section of bike path, which parallels Admiralty Way, is a very popular dog-walking spot where you'll spy an incredible array of breeds. Most owners are good about keeping their canines on a leash, but watch out for the occasional off-leash dog.

This section of bike path will cross Washington Avenue. There is a crossing signal here as well, and the button can be found on a pole at the right side of the middle ramp exiting the bike path. Cross Washington Avenue and turn left. You'll see a clearly marked bike lane that will take you to the next section of path at the end of Washington Avenue. To your

This ride has the distinction of being both the flattest ride in this guide (there is less than 150 feet of elevation gain from one end to the other) and the most endlessly entertaining.

right, you will see two paths, one marked for bicycles and another marked for pedestrians; bear left onto the bicycle path.

The next 2.5 miles of bike path are arguably some of the most interesting you will see anywhere. The path is very twisty here. You'll need to keep an eye out for people walking or cyclists stopping to look around; it can be downright crowded at times. The homes along Ocean Front Walk sport some unusual and attractive architecture, some with nautical themes. Farther along you get into the section of Venice with the shops and street vendors. This was once a very seedy area. The city of Venice has made great strides in reducing crime, going so far as to construct a police station right on the walk. Despite the changes, the area still attracts a wide variety of people. It's a popular place to view or get body art, including tattoos (both temporary and permanent) and piercings.

Weekend days you may find a drum circle. And the skateboarders are catching air any time

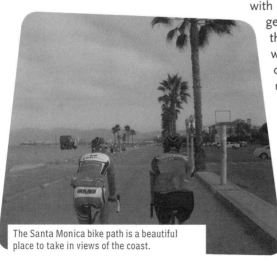

The Santa Monica bike path is a beautiful place to take in views of the coast.

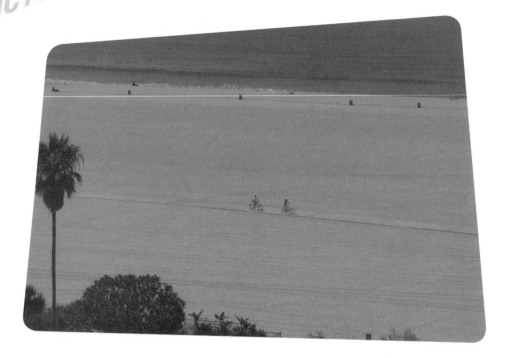

school isn't in session (and sometimes even when it is). You will also notice a large population of transient and homeless people. The shops along this stretch range from the kitschy to the weird. It's an interesting place to shop for music—and to listen to it. The Hare Krishnas jingle through daily, making the lurid scene just that much more interesting.

Athletic pursuits in addition to cycling flourish here. You'll see surfers and kids playing in the water. The handball courts are known for some very ambitious games. The street skating is good enough to warrant a picture or some video. And then there's Muscle Beach. The body builders here are huge . . . and they seem to prefer it when tourists gawk.

Should you find yourself getting peckish, the array of restaurants in the area can sate any palate, though the selection leans toward informal: burgers, dogs, pizza, and such make up the bulk. There are also many snack bars lining the bike path itself and, amazingly, many have sports drinks in addition to soft drinks.

When the path reaches the Santa Monica Pier, a tunnel takes you beneath and beyond. Although the section to the south can be a little overpopulated, the section from north of the pier to Will Rogers State Beach tends to see less action. Here is where you'll see the volleyball players, inline skaters, and joggers. How crowded these final 3 miles of path are depends entirely on the time of day and the day of the week you choose to ride here. Weekend afternoons are beyond busy.

After the Ride
With all there is to take in during the ride, it may be more fun to eat outside—with the bikes in view (locks are helpful but no guarantee)—and to watch the ever-changing scene. Put on your sunglasses, buy a cheap straw hat, and kick it.

Brentwood Star Homes Tour

Length: 20 miles

Configuration: Loop

Difficulty: Moderate

Climbing: 2,000 feet

Maximum gradient: 16%

Scenery: Landscaped yards, great architecture

Exposure: Mornings and late afternoons can be overcast

Road traffic: Moderate

Road surface: Good

Riding time: 2 hours

Maps: Los Angeles County *Thomas Guide* pages 631 and 591

In Brief

The land of the world's most infamous murder is also known as a paradise for the fabulously wealthy. Though not every home has a history leading to old-time Hollywood's leading men and ladies, these mansions are uniformly fun to check out. Set amid the canyons, the ride takes in some great hills and big-ring descents. Even if you never look at a single dwelling, the place makes for great riding.

Directions

From the I-405 and I-10 junction, travel north on the 405 and exit at Wilshire Boulevard West. After passing the Veterans' Administration hospital, move into the right lane and turn right on San Vicente. You'll quickly pass through a commercial area. After crossing Bundy, begin looking for street parking on San Vicente.

Description

The ride begins at the intersection of 26th Street and San Vicente Boulevard. Ride northeast on San Vicente; there is a wide shoulder here, plus a bike lane. Watch for drivers opening doors on your right. Just a few blocks up, turn right on South Burlingame Avenue. On your left is the exclusive Brentwood Country Club; its periphery is popular with joggers because it is much more inviting than the sidewalks of the sprawling metropolis that is LA.

Following a brief downhill, turn left at Montana Avenue. Montana will end at a T-intersection just a quarter-mile up the road; it continues to the left. A half-mile farther, turn right at Gretna Green Way. This is the street Nicole Brown Simpson was living on when she made her famous 911 call to police. Turn left on Dorothy Street and immediately left again on South Bundy Drive. To your left, at 879 South Bundy, is the site of the murders of Nicole Brown

BICYCLING

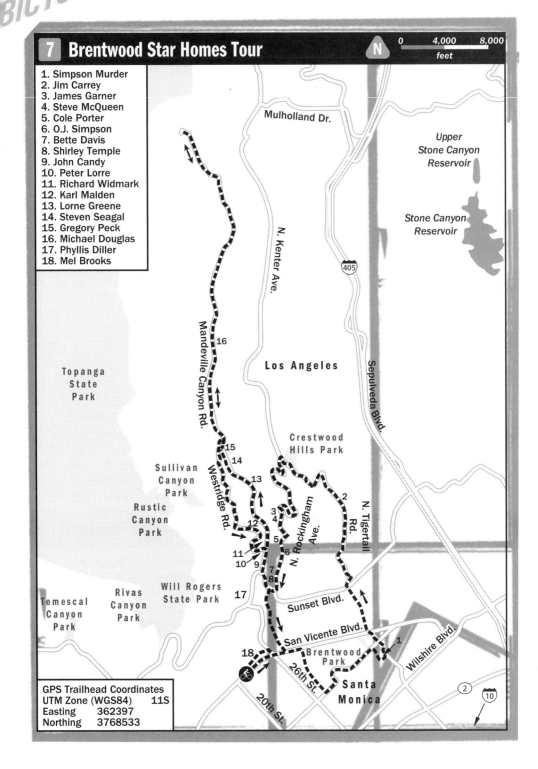

7 Brentwood Star Homes Tour

1. Simpson Murder
2. Jim Carrey
3. James Garner
4. Steve McQueen
5. Cole Porter
6. O.J. Simpson
7. Bette Davis
8. Shirley Temple
9. John Candy
10. Peter Lorre
11. Richard Widmark
12. Karl Malden
13. Lorne Greene
14. Steven Seagal
15. Gregory Peck
16. Michael Douglas
17. Phyllis Diller
18. Mel Brooks

N

0   4,000   8,000
feet

Mulholland Dr.

Upper
Stone Canyon
Reservoir

Stone Canyon
Reservoir

N. Kenter Ave.

405

Sepulveda Blvd.

Los Angeles

Topanga
State
Park

Mandeville Canyon Rd.

16

Crestwood
Hills Park

Sullivan
Canyon
Park

Westridge Rd.

15
14
13
12
11
10
9

Rustic
Canyon
Park

3
4
5
6
7
8

N. Rockingham Ave.

2

N. Tigertail Rd.

Temescal
Canyon
Park

Rivas
Canyon
Park

Will Rogers
State Park

17

Sunset Blvd.

San Vicente Blvd.

1

Wilshire Blvd.

18

Brentwood
Park

26th St.

Santa
Monica

20th St.

2

10

GPS Trailhead Coordinates
UTM Zone (WGS84)   11S
Easting   362397
Northing   3768533

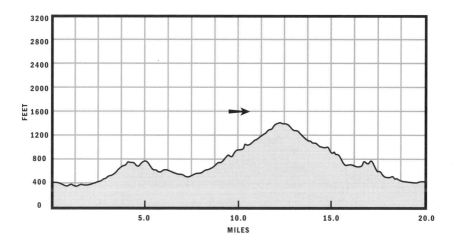

Simpson and Ron Goldman. The murder scene and consequent morbid tourist attraction resulted in the new owner's changing the address to 875 South Bundy, but it's essentially the same place.

Bundy makes a brief dogleg at San Vicente. To continue north on Bundy, turn left and then immediately right. A third of a mile up Bundy, the road becomes North Kenter Avenue. Bundy veers to the right. Continue straight on Kenter. Cross Sunset Boulevard and immediately turn right on North Tigertail Road.

Tigertail climbs immediately. The grade quickly hits 10 percent, but after 200 meters, the incline becomes much more reasonable, easing back to generally 6 or 7 percent. One mile from your turn, you will encounter Jim Carrey's house (at 615 Tigertail) on your left. As with many stars' homes, there's a gate, a wall, hedges, and not much to see.

Continue on Tigertail another 0.3 miles to Deerbrook Lane; this is the end of the first climb. Deerbrook immediately descends to your next turn, a right on Hanley Avenue.

Hanley will continue to descend for 100 yards before bending left and making a brief, twisting kick up to a T-intersection with North Kenter Avenue. Turn left onto Kenter and begin descending. There is a stop sign at Leonard Road. Be sure to stop; police are known to stake out the intersection.

You'll pass a school on your right. Turn right here onto Elkins Road, which curls behind the school. This next hill isn't long, but it is the steepest of the day. It would be easy to go too hard early and flame out before you hit the top. Downshift and be patient for the real kicker, which comes after the second left bend. Less than 100 yards on, Elkins becomes Oakmont Drive. To your right, at 33 Oakmont, is James Garner's home. Next door to him is 27 Oakmont, which was Steve McQueen's home for a number of years.

Continue downhill on Oakmont and, while viewing the stately palms that line the median, be mindful of the speed bumps. Turn right at North Rockingham Avenue. The composer Cole Porter lived at 416. At the corner of Ashford Street is

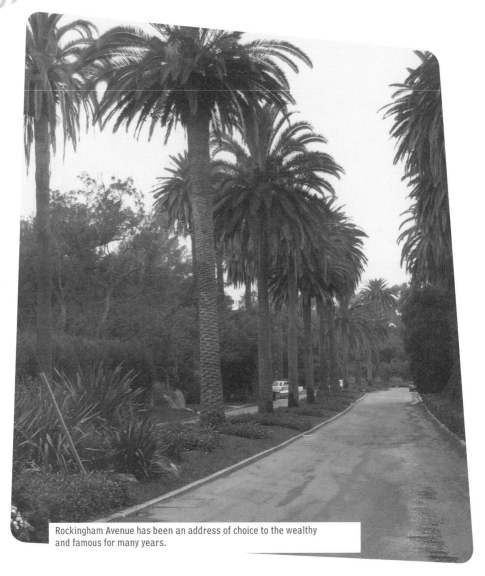

Rockingham Avenue has been an address of choice to the wealthy and famous for many years.

380 North Rockingham, which was 360 North Rockingham when it was the home of O. J. Simpson (and occasionally Kato Kaelin). After it was sold, following the civil suit, the house was razed by the new owner. Farther down the block is 301 North Rockingham, on your right, which was Bette Davis's home for many years. And a block on is 209 North Rockingham, where Shirley Temple lived until 1951.

In another hundred yards, you reach Sunset Boulevard. Sunset is very busy and very twisty (as a matter of fact, the "Dead Man's Curve" referred to in the Jan and Dean song is just over 3 miles east on Sunset—not on Mulholland, as many believe). Your route uses Sunset for a little more than 200 yards—short enough to allow you to get on and off the road between packs of cars. Wait for a pause in traffic, turn right, and big ring it down the hill. Take the very next right turn at Mandeville Canyon Road.

Mandeville Canyon has been a popular site for stars' homes for ages. While several roads spur off of Mandeville, there is just one way in or out, and that's via Mandeville Canyon Road at Sunset. This has helped keep the area private.

John Candy lived at 1630 Mandeville Canyon until his death. Peter Lorre lived at 1670 Mandeville Canyon for much of his career. Imagine having him for a neighbor! Further up on the left is Richard Widmark's home, at 1727. Another quarter-mile on is the former home of Karl Malden. Continuing north on Mandeville, the road climbs ever so slightly—a false flat of generally 2 to 3 percent. Lorne Greene's former home is on your right less than a mile farther at 2090, and another half-mile up is the former home of both Steven Seagal and Kelly LeBrock (though not at the same time) at 2282. Around the next bend is the home that was Gregory Peck's longtime residence. Halfway up the 5-mile climb, you'll pass Michael Douglas's former home at 2915 Mandeville Canyon.

The rest of the climb is just for fun. At roughly the 3200 block, the grade will increase to 4 percent and, with less than a mile to go, it will increase to 6 percent. Finally, with less than 500 yards to go, the gradient will kick up to 11 percent, just to keep you working. Because the descent isn't overly windy (not like the descents in Malibu just a few miles away), you can pedal a big gear for the whole of the decline.

Turn right at the stop sign at Chalon. Lest you get too comfortable with the descent, this is a great short climb that intersects Westridge Road, where you'll turn left. It bends a few times, but at the first sharp left bend take a moment to pull to the right and look into Sullivan Canyon. The hill directly opposite you is part of Pacific Palisades;

another ride in this guide is devoted to that area. Atop the hill is the home of the producer Norman Lear; the large parking structure with the tennis court on top is reputed to hold 24 cars . . . and isn't popular with neighbors.

Release your brakes, and you'll be treated to a brief but quick descent back to Mandeville Canyon. Turn right and, at Sunset Boulevard, turn left. Move into the right lane immediately and attack the short hill to South Rockingham Avenue. Turn right and relax. The comedienne Phyllis Diller lives at 163 South Rockingham. Bear left at the fork onto Avondale Street and turn right on San Vicente. You can either ride back to your car now or take a slight detour to see the home that Mel Brooks lives in and once shared with his wife Anne Bancroft. For a view, turn right on 21st Street and right again immediately on La Mesa Drive. Brooks's home is 2301, on the left. Continue on La Mesa to 26th Street and turn right to head to your car.

After the Ride
There are some shops and restaurants (not to mention a trendy yoga studio) at the intersection of 26th Street and San Vicente. The Brentwood Country Market is worth a walk; it's a quaint reminder of a bygone era, and Brentwood residents are very protective of it. If you'd like more selection, head east on San Vicente. Between Bundy and South Barrington Avenue are a number of great restaurants and some ritzy shopping.

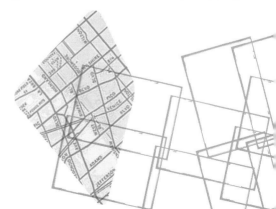

The Nicholls Canyon Ride

Length: 25 miles

Configuration: Loop

Difficulty: Difficult

Climbing: 2,000 feet

Maximum gradient: 15%

Scenery: Homes in Beverly Hills, West Hollywood, the Los Angeles Basin, and the San Fernando Valley

Exposure: Mornings can be overcast

Road traffic: Moderate, if you leave early enough

Road surface: Good, except for some spots on Nicholls Canyon and Mulholland

Riding time: 2 hours

Maps: Los Angeles County *Thomas Guide* pages 632, 592, 593, 563, 562, 561, 591, and 631

In Brief

Few rides offer the range of views that this one does. With an ever-changing orientation, riders are afforded views of Beverly Hills, Century City, West Hollywood, downtown Los Angeles, and the whole of the San Fernando Valley: the San Gabriel Mountains serve as a backdrop for views to the north. The ride along Mulholland will take you by the homes of a number of stars, though some of the biggest palaces you see are owned by successes unknown to the average person.

The course itself is difficult, with slightly more than 2,000 feet of climbing in only 25 miles. Although it can be attempted on almost any bike, you will want some low gears for the climbing, which commences with the turn onto Nicholls Canyon. All but the strongest local riders will use a 39 x 25 low gear on their road bike.

This ride is one that offers unparalleled views of the city but should be attempted only early in the morning. Traffic is simply too heavy otherwise. Roadies who like group rides have the best opportunity to do this circuit. This is a regularly occurring group ride, and riders meet at 8 a.m. on Sunday.

Directions

From I-405, exit Santa Monica Boulevard eastbound. Travel just more than a half-mile east on Santa Monica Boulevard. Turn right on Westwood Boulevard and drive two blocks to La Grange Avenue. Turn left and begin looking for street parking.

Description

Because some of the roads on this ride are heavily traveled, this route is much more enjoyable if done with the Sunday group ride. The group meets at the northeast corner of the intersection and rolls out a few minutes after 8 a.m. Should you wish to ride this on your own, you would do well

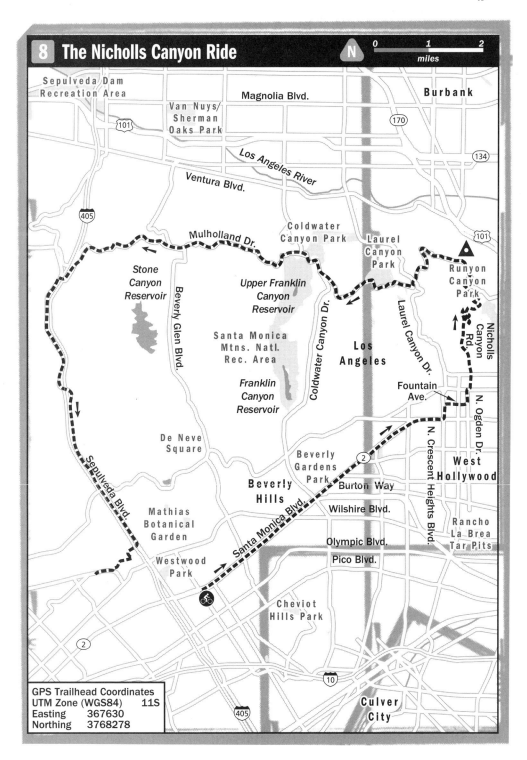

8 **The Nicholls Canyon Ride**

N

0   1   2
miles

Sepulveda Dam
Recreation Area

Magnolia Blvd.

Burbank

Van Nuys/
Sherman
Oaks Park

101

170

134

Los Angeles River

Ventura Blvd.

405

101

Mulholland Dr.

Coldwater
Canyon Park

Laurel
Canyon
Park

Runyon
Canyon
Park

Stone
Canyon
Reservoir

Beverly Glen Blvd.

Upper Franklin
Canyon
Reservoir

Coldwater Canyon Dr.

Laurel Canyon Dr.

Nicholls Canyon Rd.

Santa Monica
Mtns. Natl.
Rec. Area

**Los
Angeles**

Franklin
Canyon
Reservoir

Fountain
Ave.

N. Ogden Dr.

De Neve
Square

Sepulveda Blvd.

Beverly
Gardens
Park

2

**West
Hollywood**

N. Crescent Heights Blvd.

**Beverly
Hills**

Burton Way

Mathias
Botanical
Garden

Santa Monica Blvd.

Wilshire Blvd.

**Rancho
La Brea
Tar Pits**

Olympic Blvd.

Westwood
Park

Pico Blvd.

Cheviot
Hills Park

2

10

**Culver
City**

405

GPS Trailhead Coordinates
UTM Zone (WGS84)   11S
Easting   367630
Northing   3768278

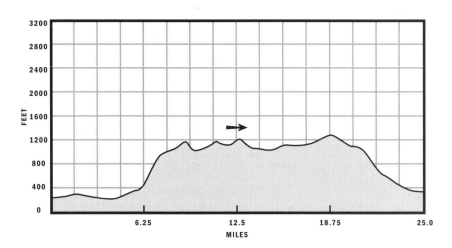

to ride on Saturday or Sunday morning and depart no later than 7 a.m.

The ride starts by heading north on Westwood Boulevard to Santa Monica Boulevard, where you turn right. Santa Monica Boulevard is a very wide road with three lanes in each direction; you will ride on Santa Monica for just over 5 miles. The view is a window on affluence, beginning with Century City. This complex is home to 20th Century Fox Studios; when the huge office mall was first completed, Fox shot *Return to the Planet of the Apes* here.

Continuing on Santa Monica Boulevard, you will enter Beverly Hills, a city whose name is synonymous with fabulous wealth. Crossing Rodeo Drive, you'll see exclusive shopping to your right. To your left are homes that most of us can only dream of entering, let alone owning. Take a moment to notice the pristine grounds; it seems there must be a city ordinance requiring everyone to have a gardener on retainer.

Santa Monica Boulevard continues into West Hollywood, which is home to many stars and a very lively gay and lesbian popu-

lation. Many of Los Angeles's most famous bars and music clubs are in this area.

Turn left at Crescent Heights Boulevard. The course will zigzag slightly to deliver you to the base of the ride's big climb. Although your ride has been almost dead flat so far, Crescent Heights will rise with a false flat. Ride two blocks on Crescent Heights, and turn right on Fountain Avenue. Ride five blocks, and turn left on North Ogden Drive, which also inclines gently. Go two blocks and turn right at Sunset Boulevard. Immediately move into the left lane and turn onto North Genessee Avenue, which becomes Nicholls Canyon Road after it crosses Hollywood Boulevard.

Nicholls Canyon Road is a narrow, two-lane road with pavement that isn't always great. From the light at Hollywood to Mulholland Drive, the climb is 3 miles and ascends 700 feet. On paper, that makes for an average gradient of 4.5 percent, though the first mile of the climb tends to be much steeper. There aren't any particularly large potholes, but the bumps can throw you off your rhythm. One mile into the climb

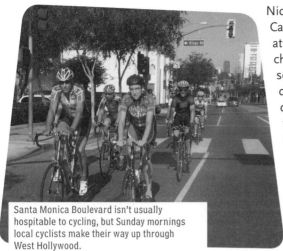

Santa Monica Boulevard isn't usually hospitable to cycling, but Sunday mornings local cyclists make their way up through West Hollywood.

there is an important turn. It will appear as if Nicholls Canyon Road goes straight, but in fact it turns right; the portion that continues straight is Jalmia Drive. Turn right and continue on Nicholls Canyon.

Following the right turn, the gradient eases up noticeably. Eventually, the road drops following one of the many right-hand switchbacks. This will give you a moment to recuperate before hitting the right turn onto Woodrow Wilson Drive, which the locals refer to as "the wall." This pitch holds a steady 15 percent and is the biggest challenge of the entire ride.

Turn left on Mulholland Drive. While the road doesn't go flat, you will be grateful for the end of the torture. If you have elected to do this ride with the group, now is the time to take stock. If you have made it up the wall with one of the small groups that formed on the climb, stay on them following the turn. If, however, you arrived at the top alone, you can take the opportunity to recover, knowing that other riders will catch you shortly.

Mulholland climbs through a series of steps as you ride west from Nicholls Canyon to Sepulveda Boulevard. The first two come in the 1.8-mile stretch between

Nicholls Canyon Road and Laurel Canyon Boulevard. There is a light at Laurel Canyon; look at it as a chance to recover. The next 2.4-mile section climbs steadily until a 90-degree right-hand bend, and then it descends through a series of bends to the intersection with Coldwater Canyon Drive. Mulholland breaks at this point. Merge right with Coldwater Canyon; the road descends to a tight left-hand turn and on to a sweeping right-hand bend. Follow the bend and move into the left-turn lane for the turn back onto Mulholland Drive.

Between Coldwater Canyon Drive and Benedict Canyon Drive, this 2.6-mile section of Mulholland climbs a little more than 200 feet.

After crossing Beverly Glen Drive, the final 1.5 miles of climbing ascends 200 feet, but half that is gained in the last half mile; if you're with a group, they will sprint for the top of the climb. Whether alone or with a group, many folks make the mistake of launching their effort immediately following the downhill, right-hand bend. Be patient and don't worry about the momentum you lose. Bends in the road hide the finish from view.

After topping out, your recovery starts immediately as Mulholland begins its decline to the Sepulveda Pass. Turn left just before the bridge that crosses I-405, and continue downhill on Rimerton Road. The road will bend right before reaching two stoplights (one for cars exiting I-405 and the other, next to it, for Sepulveda Boulevard); the lights require a short wait. A few riders usually regroup at the entrance to the Skirball Cultural Center (well worth a visit, though perhaps not in Lycra). Whether you're alone or with a group, this is a great spot to have a drink and an energy bar.

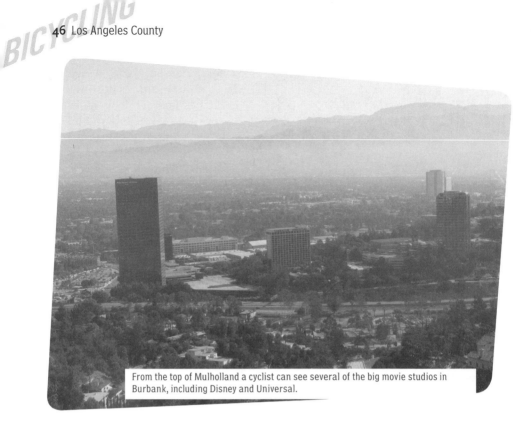

From the top of Mulholland a cyclist can see several of the big movie studios in Burbank, including Disney and Universal.

From here to the finish, the ride is essentially downhill. If you are alone, keep an eye on the traffic approaching from behind. Cars descending the Sepulveda Pass will be traveling very quickly. Groups descending have the advantage of being more visible than a single rider and will take up the right lane. After crossing the light at Montana Avenue, the group will wind up for a final sprint roughly 500 yards from the light. There is a mark on the road at about 200 yards, and the sprint coincides with a line painted on the road 150 yards from your next turn, onto Constitution Avenue.

Pass through the tunnel under I-405. You will now be on the grounds of the Veterans' Administration hospital. Almost any route you take west through the hospital's property will result in your reaching Bringham Avenue, but it will be quicker if you turn left on Bonsall Avenue, right on Grant, left on Dewey, right on Eisenhower,

and left on Bringham. The turns come quickly, less than every 100 yards. Once on Bringham, turn right on San Vicente. Riders on the group ride will turn left on Gorham and stop for coffee at the corner. It's a relaxing way to end such a strenuous ride.

If you parked near the start of the ride, you can get back there easily. Ride east on San Vicente Boulevard. It will curve right, to the south, and cross Wilshire Boulevard. At this point, San Vicente becomes Federal Avenue. Turn left onto Santa Monica Boulevard. Less than 1 mile east, turn right on Westwood, and two blocks south you will find La Grange Avenue.

After the Ride

In addition to the coffee shop where the group stops, there are a number of restaurants right in the Brentwood neighborhood where the ride ends.

9

Pacific Palisades Star Homes Tour

AT A GLANCE	**Length:** 9 miles
	Configuration: Loop
	Difficulty: Moderate
	Climbing: 750 feet

Maximum gradient: 11%

Scenery: Landscaped yards, great architecture

Exposure: Mornings and late afternoons can be overcast

Road traffic: Light

Road surface: Generally good

Riding time: 1 hour

Maps: Los Angeles County *Thomas Guide* pages 631 and 671

In Brief

Of the exclusive communities that lie at the foot of the Santa Monica Mountains, Pacific Palisades is the farthest west, situated where the mountains meet the ocean. As with the communities of Beverly Hills, Bel Air, and Brentwood, some of Hollywood's biggest stars call Pacific Palisades home. This short tour will take you by a number of homes that will wow you, whether or not they are owned by people whose names you know.

Directions

From the I-405 and I-10 junction, travel north on the 405 and exit at Wilshire Boulevard West. After passing the Veterans' Administration hospital, move into the right lane and turn right on San Vicente Boulevard. You'll pass through a small commercial area. After crossing 26th Street, begin looking for street parking on San Vicente.

Description

The ride begins at the intersection of San Vicente Boulevard and Seventh Street. Ride north on Seventh; the road will start out flat but bends to the right and turns sharply downhill. Following this bend is a sweeping left turn; set up far to the right before beginning your turn. It is important not to get too close to the yellow line; cars traveling uphill sometimes take the turn a little wide.

Before the hill flattens, turn right at West Channel Road. West Channel becomes East Channel after crossing Sage Lane. Another 100 yards on, the flat but pockmarked road turns left and uphill and becomes Amalfi Drive. The road here is narrow, and there are usually a great many cars and trucks parked on the shoulder. The road surface isn't the best either; it will be a little bumpy until you've passed the last of four switchbacks. The final switchback is the steepest, but it is mercifully short; stand up and hammer the short rise. Now the sightseeing begins.

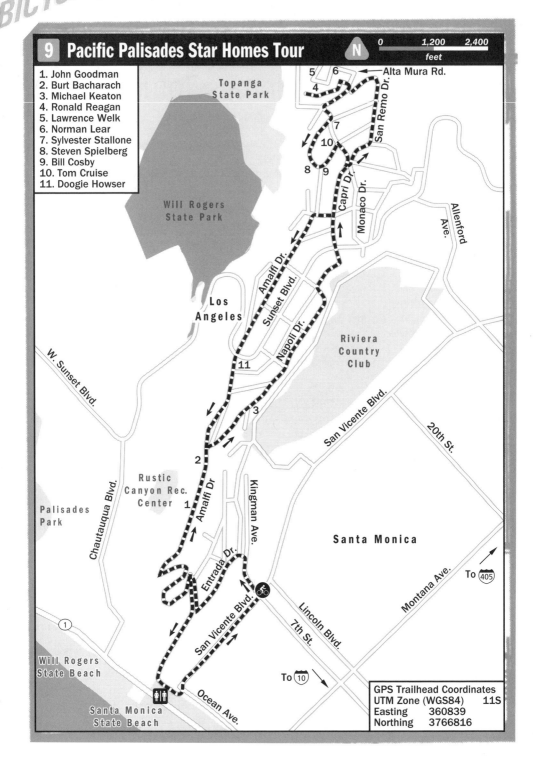

N

0   1,200   2,400
feet

1. John Goodman
2. Burt Bacharach
3. Michael Keaton
4. Ronald Reagan
5. Lawrence Welk
6. Norman Lear
7. Sylvester Stallone
8. Steven Spielberg
9. Bill Cosby
10. Tom Cruise
11. Doogie Howser

Alta Mura Rd.

Topanga State Park

San Remo Dr.

Capri Dr.

Monaco Dr.

Allenford Ave.

Will Rogers State Park

Amalfi Dr.

Sunset Blvd.

Napoli Dr.

Los Angeles

Riviera Country Club

W. Sunset Blvd.

San Vicente Blvd.

20th St.

Rustic Canyon Rec. Center

Amalfi Dr

Kingman Ave.

Santa Monica

Chautauqua Blvd.

Palisades Park

Entrada Dr.

San Vicente Blvd.

Lincoln Blvd.

7th St.

Montana Ave.

To 405

To 10

Will Rogers State Beach

Ocean Ave.

Santa Monica State Beach

GPS Trailhead Coordinates
UTM Zone (WGS84)   11S
Easting   360839
Northing   3766816

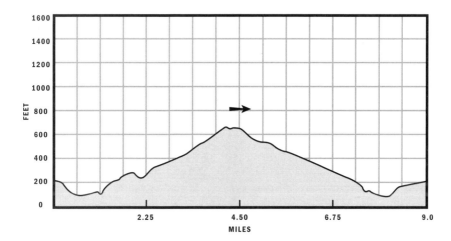

Amalfi Drive will continue to rise as a 1 to 2 percent false flat. The first point of interest you'll encounter is the former home of John Goodman, at 619 Amalfi, on the left. This home is a little unusual in that there is no gate; instead, the home is accessed via the garage. Burt Bacharach's home is 100 yards up on the left, at 681. Just beyond that, turn right on Napoli; the road will drop slightly and flatten out. Just as it begins to rise, you'll see Michael Keaton's home on your right, at 826 Napoli.

The road will continue to rise and then bend left. At Corsica Drive, turn right and immediately turn left onto Capri Drive. The very next intersection is Sunset Boulevard. If no cars are present, press the pedestrian-crossing button to change the light. One of the ironies of this neighborhood is that some of its beauty is interrupted by seemingly endless construction. Houses are constantly being torn down and replaced by buildings large enough to contain the municipal functions of a small city.

Continue on Capri to Monaco Drive and bear right. Here, the view of palm tree–lined D'Este Drive is considerably compromised by the presence of construction workers' vehicles. It's easy to conclude that all the cars here fit into one of two categories: 1990s vintage Japanese compacts and luxury land yachts you can't afford.

Monaco intersects San Remo Drive; turn left and continue uphill. San Remo then makes a sharp bend to the left and becomes Casale Drive. Immediately after that, turn right on Alta Mura Drive. The road then forks—San Onofre goes left, while Alta Mura twists uphill to the right. Do not attempt to climb Alta Mura; it is a private road, and trespassers can be fined and jailed. Lawrence Welk lived at 1694 Alta Mura for much of his career. At the top of Alta Mura is the home of the producer Norman Lear; it includes a 24-car garage, which, when constructed, was not popular with neighbors.

President Ronald Reagan lived at 1169 San Onofre from 1956 until 1980, when he moved into a much larger white home on the East Coast. Double back on San Onofre and turn right on Casale. Immediately turn left on Capri and then right, back onto Amalfi. At the southwest corner of Capri and Amalfi is a house with enormous hedges (this in a land of many enormous hedges). This home, 1570 Amalfi, was Sylvester Stallone's for many years. Continue on Amalfi to 1515; you'll know it by the hedges. This is the director Steven Spielberg's home.

Rather than continue on Amalfi, turn left onto Sorrento Drive. On the southeast corner of Amalfi and Sorrento is Bill Cosby's home. There is a plaque above the front door that says "Ennis" to commemorate the entertainer's late son. Sorrento rises slightly and then continues downhill. On the left, at 1525 (on the corner of Sorrento and Capri), is Tom Cruise's home. When crews are at work on the place, the gates will stand open and you can see a tree house up in the canopy. Looks like fun.

Descend Capri to Romany Drive and turn right. At Amalfi, turn left and descend back to Sunset. Once again, use the pedestrian crossing if no cars are present. Immediately after crossing Sunset, you can see the house used for the exterior shots of the home in *Doogie Howser, MD,* at 796 Amalfi, on the left.

Your descent will take you back by Burt Bacharach's home and John Goodman's former home. As you reach the series of switchbacks, the first steep (though short) part of the descent ends at a stop sign. It's a good idea to be very careful at this intersection; many local residents fail to stop.

Because of the questionable state of the road along this stretch and the fact that construction crews are always at work at one address or another, bombing this descent isn't a great idea; it's a real wasted opportunity. Cross at the light at Entrada, (it will seem like you are going straight) and climb Ocean Avenue Extended. This is a much gentler

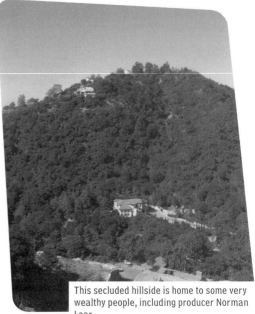

This secluded hillside is home to some very wealthy people, including producer Norman Lear.

climb than the Seventh Street ascent. At the top, the road bends left and you will see public restrooms on your right. Just beyond the restrooms, move into the left lane and turn onto San Vicente. The long median means that, to get back to your car, you will have to ride a block or two beyond your car and turn at one of the median pass-throughs.

After the Ride
On San Vicente, between Bundy Drive and South Barrington Avenue, are some great restaurants and ritzy shopping. Alternatively, take Seventh Street to Montana Avenue to reach Santa Monica's trendy heart. If you'd like to take a hike up in the Santa Monica Mountains, visit Will Rogers State Park; its entrance can be reached by turning right on Will Rogers State Park Road from Sunset Boulevard. You'll pass Arnold Schwarzenegger's former compound at the intersection of Sunset Boulevard and Evans Road (don't drive on Evans; it is a private road).

10 Beverly Hills Star Homes Loop

AT A GLANCE

Length: 22 miles (also 6-mile option)
Configuration: Loop
Difficulty: Moderate (shortcut is easy)
Climbing: 2,500 feet

Maximum gradient: 10%

Scenery: Stunning homes, gorgeous landscaping, precipitous overlooks

Exposure: Almost no shade

Road traffic: Light except on Wilshire and Sunset

Road surface: Mostly good

Riding time: 2.5 hours

Maps: Los Angeles County *Thomas Guide* pages 592 and 632

In Brief

Even without a list of the stars whose homes you are viewing, this ride affords you views of spectacular opulence and consumption on a scale many of us can't fathom, and most of us can't help but envy the homeowners. The first few miles are very easy and offer riders an opportunity to return to the start before encountering the big hills or the busy streets; this early portion is perfect for riders with mountain bikes or cruisers who want a shorter, gentler ride. For those looking for some hills, a few fun descents, and the biggest, most impressive estates, the ride gains momentum with each mile. The homes may have beckoned you here, but the terrain will bring you back for more.

Directions

Exit I-405 at Sunset Boulevard East. Drive 4 miles to Will Rogers Park at North Canon Drive, and look for parking. The parking here is free, and there is usually plenty of space.

Description

Few communities in the world are as associated with success as Beverly Hills is. Thanks to such shows as *The Beverly Hillbillies* and *Beverly Hills 90210*, much of the world thinks of Beverly Hills as a place far removed from the life of the ordinary man. Beginning with the purchase of a plot of land on Summit Drive in 1919 by Douglas Fairbanks and Mary Pickford, Beverly Hills became the hometown of Hollywood stars. Since then, most great cinematic stars have had at least one address in this community of 35,000.

Your ride begins smack dab in the middle of one of Beverly Hills's richest neighborhoods, at Will Rogers Park. Rogers, a political humorist, was one of the town's earliest boosters. Because there are so many homes of interest, the addresses will be listed by waypoint number at the end. You can then choose when and where you wish to stop. Most homes are right on the

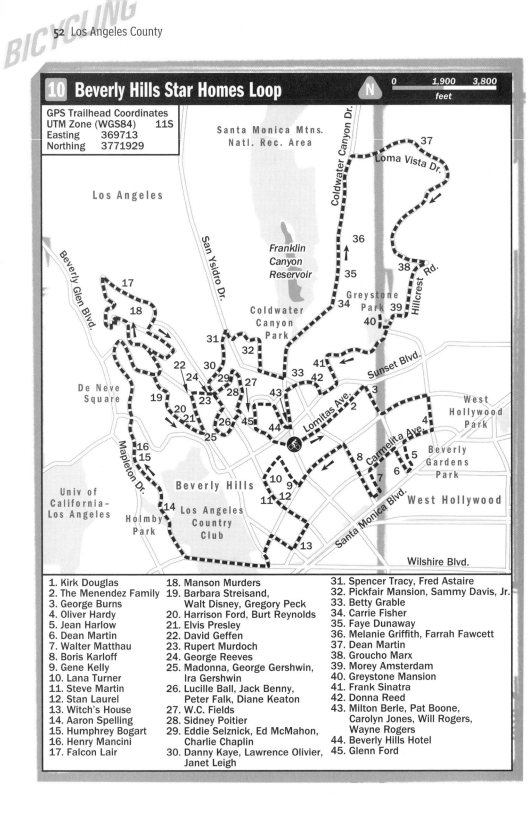

10 Beverly Hills Star Homes Loop

N

0   1,900   3,800
feet

GPS Trailhead Coordinates
UTM Zone (WGS84)   11S
Easting   369713
Northing   3771929

Santa Monica Mtns.
Natl. Rec. Area

Coldwater Canyon Dr.

Los Angeles

San Ysidro Dr.

Franklin
Canyon
Reservoir

Loma Vista Dr.   37

36

35

38   Hillcrest Rd.

Greystone
Park   39

Coldwater
Canyon
Park

34   40

Beverly Glen Blvd.

17

18

31

32

33

41   Sunset Blvd.

42

22   30   29   27   43   3

24   28   2

De Neve
Square   19   23   26   45   44   Lomitas Ave.   West
Hollywood
Park

20   21   25

16   15   4   Beverly
Gardens
Park

Mapleton Dr.   8   Carmelita Ave.   5

7   6

Univ of
California–
Los Angeles   Beverly Hills   10   9   West Hollywood

Holmby
Park   14   Los Angeles
Country
Club   11   12   Santa Monica Blvd.

13

Wilshire Blvd.

1. Kirk Douglas
2. The Menendez Family
3. George Burns
4. Oliver Hardy
5. Jean Harlow
6. Dean Martin
7. Walter Matthau
8. Boris Karloff
9. Gene Kelly
10. Lana Turner
11. Steve Martin
12. Stan Laurel
13. Witch's House
14. Aaron Spelling
15. Humphrey Bogart
16. Henry Mancini
17. Falcon Lair

18. Manson Murders
19. Barbara Streisand,
     Walt Disney, Gregory Peck
20. Harrison Ford, Burt Reynolds
21. Elvis Presley
22. David Geffen
23. Rupert Murdoch
24. George Reeves
25. Madonna, George Gershwin,
     Ira Gershwin
26. Lucille Ball, Jack Benny,
     Peter Falk, Diane Keaton
27. W.C. Fields
28. Sidney Poitier
29. Eddie Selznick, Ed McMahon,
     Charlie Chaplin
30. Danny Kaye, Lawrence Olivier,
     Janet Leigh

31. Spencer Tracy, Fred Astaire
32. Pickfair Mansion, Sammy Davis, Jr.
33. Betty Grable
34. Carrie Fisher
35. Faye Dunaway
36. Melanie Griffith, Farrah Fawcett
37. Dean Martin
38. Groucho Marx
39. Morey Amsterdam
40. Greystone Mansion
41. Frank Sinatra
42. Donna Reed
43. Milton Berle, Pat Boone,
     Carolyn Jones, Will Rogers,
     Wayne Rogers
44. Beverly Hills Hotel
45. Glenn Ford

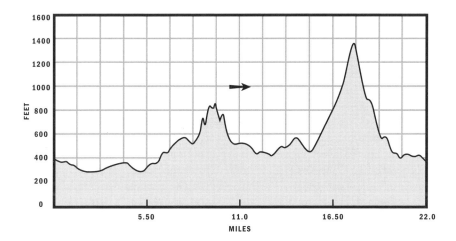

route, but some will require a brief detour. One caveat: stars move nearly as often as migrant farm workers or Canada geese— even so-called current addresses could be two addresses out of date! The homes listed definitely belonged to the stars in question at some point, however.

From the intersection of North Cañon Drive, North Beverly Drive, and Lomitas Avenue, ride northeast on Lomitas. Continue to North Maple Drive and turn right. Ride one block south on North Maple and turn left on Elevado Avenue. You'll notice that this part of Beverly Hills is on just enough of a slope to make you work a bit and allow you some nice chances to coast.

Turn right on North Alta Drive. One block down, turn left on Carmelita Avenue. Ride three blocks and turn left on Maple Drive. At the next intersection, turn left down the frontage road that parallels Santa Monica Boulevard. Immediately after the alley, turn right onto North Elm Drive. Pedal up the slight grade past Carmelita to Elevado Avenue, then turn left. This stretch of road will give a truly impressive view of Beverly Hills. Once on Elevado, go four blocks to North Rodeo Drive and turn right. Again, you'll be headed slightly uphill. At the next intersection, turn left on Lomitas Avenue and spin the two blocks to North Bedford Drive. Turn left and coast downhill to Carmelita. Turn right and head three blocks down to Walden Drive, where you'll turn right again.

At the intersection of Walden Drive and Elevado Avenue, you have a choice to make. Those on beach cruisers and mountain bikes might prefer to go straight and turn right at Lomitas Drive to go back to the start. Certainly, for anyone on a bike short on low gears or anyone who dislikes heavier traffic, this is an appropriate opportunity to finish. Those unperturbed by hills and traffic should turn left on Elevado and take it to Wilshire Boulevard.

Most daylight hours of most days, Wilshire is too busy to ride comfortably. If you undertake this ride on a weekend morning, you'll find an acceptable level of traffic for your short (half-mile) stint on this road. Turn right on Comstock Avenue. Your course for nearly the next 2 miles is uphill; downshift and settle in for the climb. Bear right at Club View Drive, and soon after, turn right onto South Mapleton Drive. At Sunset Boulevard, South Mapleton changes to North Mapleton Drive. Almost immediately after crossing Sunset, bear right on North Faring Road. As Faring bends around Westlake School, it becomes Brooklawn Drive and heads downhill briefly.

Turn left on Angelo Drive and resume climbing. This next 1.25 miles is the steepest, most significant hill thus far. The hill will at times reach a 9-percent grade and will twist up some slight switchbacks. The remoteness of the area and terrain don't seem very Beverly Hills—perhaps one of the most surprising things about this course. Turn right on Davies Drive and follow a sharp hairpin onto Cielo Drive. Follow the spur up Bella Drive; this is one home you must see—Rudolph Valentino's Falcon Lair. Consider the fact that this was built *before* the Great Depression and that it is big by any standards, even today's. Continue down

Cielo Drive and turn right on Shadybrook. Shadybrook heads up a small hill, and becomes Hillgrove Drive, then Maybrook Drive, which has yet another hill.

At Angelo Drive, turn left. This short stretch of road will look familiar; you were here minutes ago heading the other way. This time, however, when Angelo reaches North Carolwood Drive, turn left and follow it for a short flat before you descend. Watch for the left turn on Ladera Drive. It's easy to miss the nearly hairpin turn. Bear left on Bridle Lane, which intersects Angelo Drive almost immediately. Turn right and pedal on to Benedict Canyon Drive, a fairly major street coming down from Mulholland; watch for descending cars. Turn right only two blocks down at North Roxbury Drive. Roxbury curves to the left; just as it straightens out, turn left on Lexington Road.

Cross Benedict Canyon and immediately turn left on Hartford Way, then immediately right on Cove Way. When Cove intersects Summit Drive, turn left and follow it downhill to your last visit to Benedict Canyon.

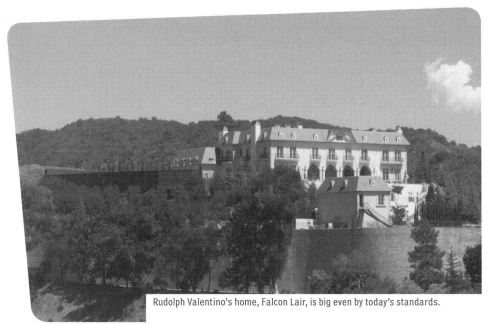

Rudolph Valentino's home, Falcon Lair, is big even by today's standards.

Turn right onto Benedict Canyon and right again at your next opportunity, at San Ysidro Drive. A half-mile up the hill, turn right onto Pickfair Way; here the hill tops out. Make an immediate left on Marilyn Drive and another left on Laurel Way for a brief downhill that takes you into the final and longest climb of the ride.

Laurel Way intersects North Beverly Drive. Turn left and begin the 2.7-mile, 900-foot climb up Coldwater Canyon Drive and Cherokee Lane—a nearly 7-percent gradient. Climb Coldwater 1.8 miles. Cherokee is to your right, and after the turn you climb another 0.9 miles. Shortly after the turn, Cherokee becomes Loma Vista Drive. After you make it over this hill, there are four small hills on your way back to the car.

Be careful not to build up too great a head of steam on the descent or you'll miss your next turn, a left onto Dabney Lane, only 0.8 miles into the downhill. The road kicks up briefly and then resumes its descent once you turn right on North Hillcrest Road. Again, watch your speed as you approach your next turn, a half-mile on. Turn right onto Drury Lane and break for your left turn back onto Loma Vista Drive. Watch for both uphill and downhill traffic here. Immediately after entering the lane, watch for the steep driveway on your right that leads to Greystone Park—it's so worth climbing it for the view. Watch the channels in the concrete as you turn.

Head back down Greystone's driveway, watching the channels in the concrete as you enter the road. The intersection you reach 100 feet later is rather broad and open. Bear slightly right onto Doheny Road. Your course here is largely downhill, with two hills remaining. Doheny bends to the left and becomes Foothill Road. Follow it down to Sunset. Turn right onto Sunset, follow it one block to Lexington Road, and turn right. This gets you back off Sunset and on the hill up to North Beverly Drive. Turn left, drop back to Sunset, and immediately make the hairpin turn onto North Crescent Drive for your final kick uphill. Turn left onto Lexington one last time and immediately left again onto Oxford Way, where you can coast at last. Oxford quickly becomes Hartford Way and ends at Sunset. Cross Sunset to Will Rogers Park.

After the Ride

Even if you're not rich enough to be a world-class consumer (and you're not, or you would already be living in Beverly Hills), take the time to wander the shops on Rodeo Drive. There are a number of great restaurants, not to mention boutiques that could inspire you to spend your children's college fund, or your inheritance. Or both. You might consider getting your lunch to go and driving up North Beverly Drive to Franklin Canyon Reservoir. The park there is a stunning throwback amid the new development.

Waypoints

1. **Kirk Douglas**—805 North Rexford Drive; his current home
2. **Marlene Dietrich**—822 North Rexford Drive; her former home
3. **Menendez Family**—722 North Elm Drive; brothers Lyle and Erik murdered their parents here
4. **Ivan Reitman**—704 North Elm Drive
5. **George Burns**—720 North Maple Drive; his last home
6. **Barbara Stanwyck**—718 North Hillcrest Drive
7. **Spike Jones**—708 North Oakhurst Drive
8. **Oliver Hardy**—612 North Alta Drive
9. **Jean Harlow**—512 North Palm Drive
10. **Dean Martin**—511 North Maple Drive; his first home in Beverly Hills

11. **Walter Matthau**—516 Alpine Drive; his first home in Beverly Hills

12. **Boris Karloff**—629 North Rexford Drive

13. **Jimmy Durante**—511 North Beverly Drive; his final home

14. **Carl Reiner**—714 North Rodeo Drive

15. **Gene Kelly**—725 North Rodeo Drive

16. **Lana Turner**—730 North Bedford Drive; one of her former homes

17. **Mia Farrow**—809 North Roxbury Drive

18. **Steve Martin**—721 North Bedford Drive; one of his former homes

19. **Stan Laurel**—718 North Bedford Drive

20. **Clara Bow**—512 North Bedford Drive; the original "it" girl

21. **Witch's House**—516 North Walden Avenue; used in silent films of the 1920s

22. **Aaron Spelling**—594 Mapleton Drive; 123-room mansion

23. **Playboy Mansion**—10236 Charing Cross Road; site of the reality show and infamous parties

24. **Jack Benny**—10231 Charing Cross Road; his last home in Beverly Hills

25. **Humphrey Bogart**—232 Mapleton Drive; the site of many Rat Pack gatherings

26. **Henry Mancini**—216 South Mapleton Drive; one of his former homes

27. **Sonny and Cher**—364 St. Cloud Road; one of their former homes

28. **Johnny Carson**—400 St. Cloud Road; occupied by a former wife

29. **Ronald Reagan**—668 St. Cloud Road; the home he retired to after his presidency

30. **Rudolph Valentino**—1436 Bella Drive; Falcon Lair couldn't keep his fans out

31. **Site of the Manson Murders**—10066 Cielo Drive

32. **Gregory Peck**—375 Carolwood Drive

33. **Walt Disney**—355 Carolwood Drive

34. **Barbara Streisand**—301 Carolwood Drive; one of her former homes

35. **Jennifer Anniston**—1026 Ridgedale Drive; one of her former homes

36. **George Harrison, Dan Rowan, and Burt Reynolds**—245 Carolwood Drive; a former home of each entertainer

37. **Elvis Presley**—144 Monovale Drive; his last home in Beverly Hills

38. **Haderway Hall**—10000 Sunset Boulevard; site of nearly a dozen statues

39. **Gene Hackman**—9901 Copley Drive

40. **Paul Newman**—907 Whittier Drive

41. **David Geffen**—1801 Angelo Drive; $47.5-million estate owned by the richest man in Hollywood

42. **Rupert Murdoch**—1330 Angelo Drive; one of the News Corp. CEO's many homes

43. **Ira Gershwin**—1021 Roxbury Drive; moved to this house after George's death

44. **Diane Keaton**—1015 North Roxbury Drive

45. **Ira and George Gershwin**—1019 Roxbury Drive; lived in this house together until George's death; later owned by Jose Ferrer and his wife Rosemary Clooney

46. **Peter Falk**—1004 Roxbury Drive

47. **Madonna**—1015 Roxbury Street; one of her many former homes

48. **Jack Benny**—1002 Roxbury Drive; his home in the 1940s, 1950s, and 1960s

49. **Lucille Ball**—1000 Roxbury Drive; her last home

50. **Jimmy Stewart**—918 Roxbury Drive; his last home; it was torn down by the current owner

51. **W. C. Fields**—1000 Cove Way

52. **Buster Keaton**—1018 Pamela Drive

53. **Sidney Poitier**—107 Cove Way; one of his former homes

54. **Charlie Chaplin**—1085 Summit Drive; the "Breakaway House," so called because of studio carpenters' shoddy work

55. **Eddie Selznick and Ed McMahon**—1050 Summit Drive; former home for both the producer and the entertainer

56. **Green Acres**—1740 Green Acres Drive; Harold Lloyd's 40,000-sq.-ft. home for 40 years

57. **Ingrid Bergman**—1220 Benedict Canyon Road

58. **Jay Leno**—1151 Tower Road; a former home

59. **Jack Lemmon**—1143 Tower Road; a former home

60. **Bill Cosby, Michael Landon, and Bernie Brillstein**—1162 Tower Road; owned by each at different times

61. **Spencer Tracy**—1158 Tower Road; a former home

62. **Elton John**—1400 Tower Grove; one of his former homes

63. **Fred Astair**—1155 San Ysidro Drive; his last home

64. **Bruce Springsteen**—Tower Lane

65. **Danny Kaye**—1103 San Ysidro Drive; his last home

66. **George Reeves**—1579 Benedict Canyon Drive; the home where he committed suicide

67. **Laurence Olivier and Vivien Leigh**—1107 San Ysidro Drive; former home for both stars

68. **Pickfair**—1143 Summit Drive; the home Mary Pickford and Douglas Fairbanks built that began the stars' influx to Beverly Hills; the original home was torn down by Pia Zadora

69. **Sammy Davis Jr.**— 1151 Summit Drive; his last home

70. **Samuel Goldwyn**—1200 Laurel Lane

71. **Betty Grable**—1008 North Beverly Drive

72. **Carrie Fisher**—1700 Coldwater Canyon Road

73. **Faye Dunaway**—1435 Lindacrest Drive

74. **James Woods**—1520 Gilcrest Drive

75. **Melanie Griffith**—9555 Heather Road

76. **Farrah Fawcett**—9507 Heather Road

77. **Dean Martin**—2002 Loma Vista Drive; his last home

78. **Elvis Presley**—1174 Hillcrest Drive; purchased just after his marriage to Priscilla

79. **Danny Thomas**—1187 Hillcrest Drive

80. **Groucho Marx**—1083 Hillcrest Drive

81. **Morey Amsterdam**—1012 Hillcrest Drive

82. **Albert I. Brocculi**—809 Hillcrest Drive

83. **Greystone**—905 Loma Vista Drive; 55-room mansion built by oilman Edward Doheny in 1923

84. **Merv Griffin**—603 North Doheny Drive; former home

85. **Frank Sinatra**—915 Foothill Drive; his last home

86. **Donna Reed**—929 North Alpine Drive

87. **Mickey Rooney**—919 North Rexford Drive

88. **Will Rogers**—925 North Beverly Drive; home in Beverly Hills before he moved to Pacific Palisades

89. **Wayne Rogers**—916 North Beverly Drive

90. **Carolyn Jones**—907 North Beverly Drive; Morticia on the *Adam's Family*

91. **Pat Boone**—904 North Beverly Drive; his current home

92. **Beverly Hills Hotel**—9641 Sunset Boulevard; has hosted many of the richest and most famous

93. **Milton Berle**—904 North Crescent Drive; former home

94. **Milton Berle**—908 North Crescent Drive; another former home

95. **Glen Ford**—911 Oxford Way

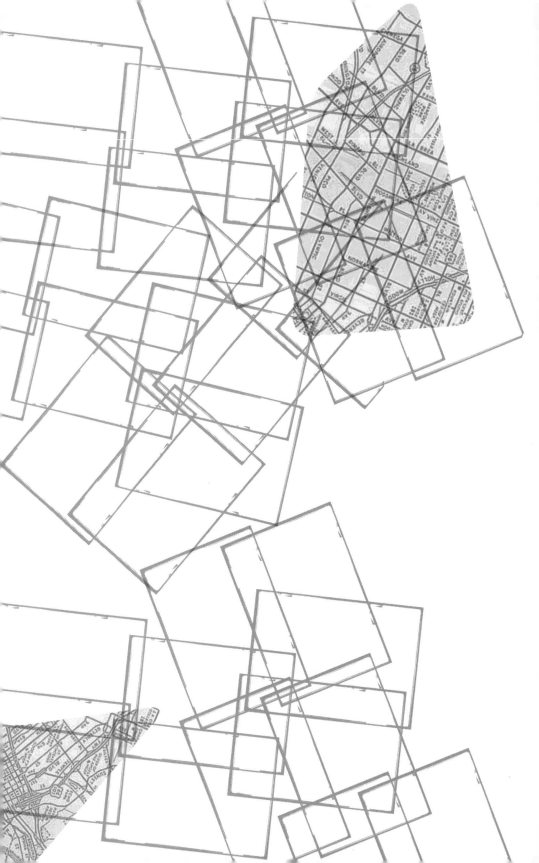

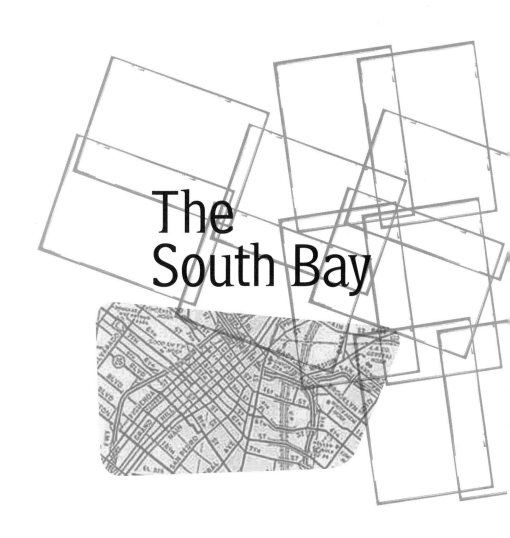

The
South Bay

11

South Bay Beach Bike Path

AT A GLANCE

Length: 11.5 miles (one way)

Configuration: Out-and-back

Difficulty: Easy

Climbing: 200 feet

Maximum gradient: 4%

Scenery: Beach, ocean, stunning homes, surfers galore, plenty of volleyball, and the cliffs of Palos Verdes

Exposure: Mornings and late afternoons can be overcast

Road traffic: Very light

Road surface: Excellent

Riding time: 1 hour

Maps: Los Angeles County *Thomas Guide* pages 702, 732, 762, and 792

In Brief

The South Bay Beach Bike Path offers the longest continuous stretch of coastal bike path in Los Angeles.

Directions

From points north: Take CA 90 West from I-405 North, and exit at Culver Boulevard. Turn left and take Culver southwest 2 miles to Vista Del Mar. It will appear that Culver bears left at the light; that is, in fact, Vista Del Mar. Bear right to continue on Culver. Turn right on Pacific Avenue and begin looking for street parking. Pacific Avenue dead-ends at the bridge.

From points south: Exit I-405 North at Crenshaw Boulevard and turn left onto 182nd Street. Immediately turn left onto Crenshaw. Travel 2 miles south on Crenshaw to Torrance Boulevard and turn right. Take Torrance 3.5 miles west to the entrance to the Redondo Beach Pier. There is parking on three levels. If you park on the

middle deck, you will be on the same level as the bike path as it passes through the pier area. Limited free parking can be found in the neighborhood to the east.

From points east: Take I-105 West to its end at Imperial Highway. Continue west on Imperial 1.75 miles to the entrance to Dockweiler Beach State Park.

Bike Rental

Visitors to Los Angeles can rent bicycles at three locations along the path.

Description

The southern end of the South Bay Beach Bike Path lies in Torrance in a tiny triangle of beach that separates Redondo Beach and Palos Verdes Estates. South of the Redondo Beach Pier, the bike path hugs the hillside often more than 50 feet below the street, which means riders on the bike path have little sense of nearby traffic.

Restrooms are plentiful on the bike

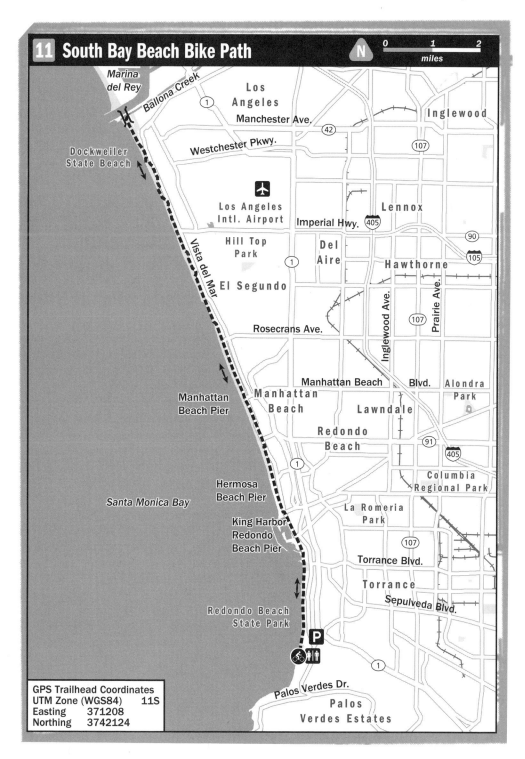

11 **South Bay Beach Bike Path**

N

0   1   2
miles

Marina
del Rey

Ballona Creek

Los
Angeles

1

Manchester Ave.

42

Inglewood

Westchester Pkwy.

107

Dockweiler
State Beach

Los Angeles
Intl. Airport

Imperial Hwy.

405

Lennox

90

Hill Top
Park

1

Del
Aire

105

Hawthorne

El Segundo

Vista del Mar

Rosecrans Ave.

107

Inglewood Ave.

Prairie Ave.

Manhattan Beach

Blvd.

Alondra
Park

Manhattan
Beach Pier

Manhattan
Beach

Lawndale

Redondo
Beach

91

405

Santa Monica Bay

Hermosa
Beach Pier

King Harbor
Redondo
Beach Pier

1

Columbia
Regional Park

La Romeria
Park

107

Torrance Blvd.

Torrance

Redondo Beach
State Park

P

Sepulveda Blvd.

🚲 🚹🚺

Palos Verdes Dr.

1

GPS Trailhead Coordinates
UTM Zone (WGS84)   11S
Easting   371208
Northing   3742124

Palos
Verdes Estates

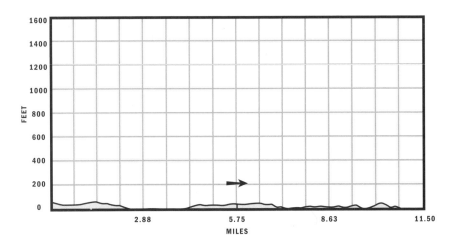

path, rarely more than a mile apart and sometimes as close as 100 yards apart. Some of the restrooms occupy buildings that also feature snack bars.

Because this section of beach is so far south, it tends not to be as busy as some of the sections of beach in Hermosa and at Manhattan Beach. Because there is a walking path adjacent to the bike path, this stretch is very popular with joggers and walkers. It is not uncommon for people to walk or jog in the bike path, so watch out for them and let them know you're approaching.

The Redondo Beach Pier is the largest of the pier developments in the South Bay. As you approach the pier, you will notice signs informing you to dismount. It can seem silly—being asked to walk your bike on a bike path—but the Redondo Beach Police mean business and are known to ticket cyclists for infractions. In the afternoon, being off the bike is helpful; many children and families are oblivious to recreating cyclists.

If you've never seen the Redondo Beach Pier, this is a great opportunity to look around. There are a number of restaurants here (not to mention an ice cream parlor) and lots of open-air seating. This is also a popular fishing spot; wander out a bit and you'll see families teaching their kids what fishing is all about. Downstairs at the harbor level are more restaurants, an arcade, and several fish markets, should you wish to purchase some fresh seafood (say, at the end of your ride).

You can remount your bicycle inside the parking structure after passing through the primary pedestrian walk. The bike path is bordered by a chain on each side. The path then turns to parallel the parking structure and overlook a portion of King Harbor. The bike path will end at North Harbor Drive. Cross North Harbor and continue north in the bike lane 0.6 miles to Yacht Club Way.

Turn left and follow the bike lane left up onto the bike path. This intersection can get a little crowded, so a touch of patience and caution is advised. The path will immediately turn right to parallel the coast once again. This is the Hermosa Beach Strand. The homes here go for millions and millions.

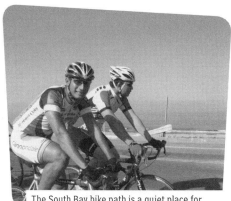

The South Bay bike path is a quiet place for rides with friends.

At this point few of the old-style beach bungalows remain: those modest digs have been replaced by mansions that may have more than 5,000 square feet of living space and are graced with enormous windows that capitalize on their stunning views.

The Hermosa Beach Pier is another popular fishing spot and a great place to take a low-key stroll and watch the surfers. Offshore winds tend to blow out the waves in the afternoon, so if you want to see impressive wave maneuvers head out for your ride in the morning. Pier Plaza, just east of the bike path, is another spot with popular restaurants and a couple of very popular bars. If you're single and want to check out the beach bar scene, come back in the late afternoon for happy hour.

On popular beach-going days, a series of red flashers mounted on light poles may be on. These lights signal riders to dismount because of the amount of foot traffic. The path in Hermosa Beach is considered multiple use, rather than exclusively for cyclists. The section with flashers is short, and there's enough to see you may wish to dismount anyway. As with the other rides in this guide, mornings are less busy; come early if you wish to ride straight through.

Our route takes us right at 24th Street, but if you were a viewer of *Beverly Hills 90210,* you may want to take a look at the beach house used in many episodes; it's at 3500 The Strand. The home is at the northern end of the Hermosa section of the bike path. Riders turn right before this point to avoid having to take the stairs next to the house. You may recognize the blue home with white trim from other Hollywood films.

At the top of the ramp up 24th Street, turn left and follow the bike lane that parallels Hermosa Avenue. The bike path will resume at Neptune Avenue when you enter Manhattan Beach. You will notice a drop in pedestrian traffic in Manhattan Beach, thanks to the footpath that parallels the bike path immediately east of it.

Manhattan Beach occupies a steep hillside, which gives many restaurants and even more homes views to kill for (OK, maybe not kill). The Manhattan Beach Pier extends into the ocean at the bottom of Manhattan Beach Boulevard. The street is very steep (a 15-percent incline) and is lined with restaurants and shops. Should you wish to avoid the hill, there is a snack bar at the end of the pier. The area north of the pier and extending to the neighborhood of El Porto at the northern end of Manhattan Beach is ground zero for beach volleyball and surfing. This section of beach hosts some of the biggest annual competitions in both sports, and any day of the week you can see their stars practicing their skills.

The South Bay Beach Bike Path offers the longest continuous stretch of coastal bike path in Los Angeles.

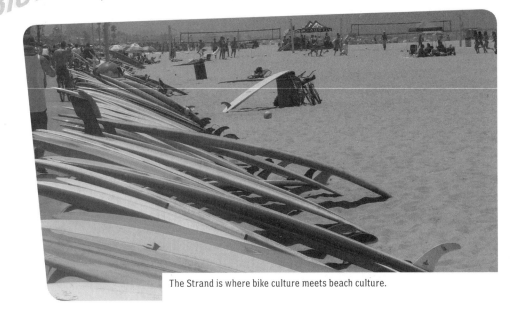

The Strand is where bike culture meets beach culture.

The path will veer away from the parking lot in El Porto and curl around a chain-link fence that separates it from the Chevron refinery. North of the refinery, you enter El Segundo. The beaches here are less populated and generally more popular with families having a day out barbecuing. After passing a parking lot, you will round a blind turn and ascend a short rise. At the top of the rise, it is possible to take a brief hang-gliding lesson. The flights are short, but the drop to the beach is said to be thrilling.

Dockweiler Beach State Park features an unlikely sight, a motor coach campground. It is nearly always full and, judging from the elaborate installations of some of the residents, it would appear that some of them are there for months at a time.

As you continue north, the beach will grow less populated. Eventually, you will pass under the flight path of planes taking off from Los Angeles International Airport. Because of the number of transcontinental and intercontinental flights originating in Los Angeles, you are likely to experience the thunder of a Boeing 747 flying overhead. Watching one take off is a thrill.

Dockweiler Beach State Park extends from El Segundo to Playa Del Rey, the northern end of the bike path. For more than a mile, the path has meandered through the sand on its own, isolated from development or homes. Bordered on both sides by sand, the concrete ribbon is at its most peaceful here. Following a bend to the right, the path cuts inland and makes a left onto the bridge over Ballona Creek. For information on what lies to the north, read the chapter on the Santa Monica Beach Bike Path (page 32).

After the Ride

If you choose to wait until after your ride is over to get a bite, there are three excellent spots to hunt for a meal and enjoy other activities. Manhattan Beach, Hermosa Beach, and Redondo Beach all offer lively options. If you parked at the north end of the path, there are a few choices nearby, but it is a short drive south on Vista Del Mar into Manhattan Beach for more selection.

12 The Donut Ride

AT A GLANCE

Length: 35 miles

Configuration: Loop

Difficulty: Moderate (solo), difficult (group)

Climbing: 2,000 feet (3,500 feet with the post loop)

Maximum gradient: 10%

Scenery: Ocean, stunning homes, cliffs, the port of Los Angeles

Exposure: Mornings are frequently overcast

Road traffic: Moderate, provided you leave early enough

Road surface: Good, except in Portuguese Bend

Riding time: 3 hours (2.5 hours with the group)

Maps: Los Angeles County *Thomas Guide* pages 792, 822, 823, 853, 854, 824, and 793

In Brief

The Donut Ride is an institution in South Bay cycling culture. The ride dates to 1973 and has maintained a reputation for being both beautiful and challenging. It draws many of the region's fastest riders (when they aren't racing). Over the years, it has attracted a Tour de France stage winner, an Olympic Gold Medalist, and more than a few national champions as regular participants. This is a consistently hilly route that will challenge you to climb well and still maintain horsepower on the flat. Without the group, the climbs won't hurt quite so badly, but it will be important to get an early start to avoid the traffic that picks up through the day.

Directions

This ride begins in south Redondo Beach in a neighborhood known as Hollywood Riviera. To get there, exit I-405 at Hawthorne Boulevard southbound. Hawthorne inter-sects I-405 south of Los Angeles International Airport and I-105, and west of I-110. Drive 5.2 miles south on Hawthorne until you reach the Pacific Coast Highway (PCH). There, turn right, drive 1.4 miles, and turn left onto Avenue I. Immediately turn left again onto South Elena Avenue. At the southwest corner of South Elena Avenue and Avenida Del Norte is a large, metered parking lot. If you prefer free parking, you can usually find some on one of the neighborhood's side streets.

Description

People meet for the Donut Ride at 8 a.m. on Saturday. Most folks arrive a little early and get coffee at one of the two coffee shops at the start of the ride. The Donut Ride got its name because it used to start at a doughnut shop in the shopping center. The doughnut shop has long since closed, but you know what they say about old habits. The group rolls out at 8:10 a.m.

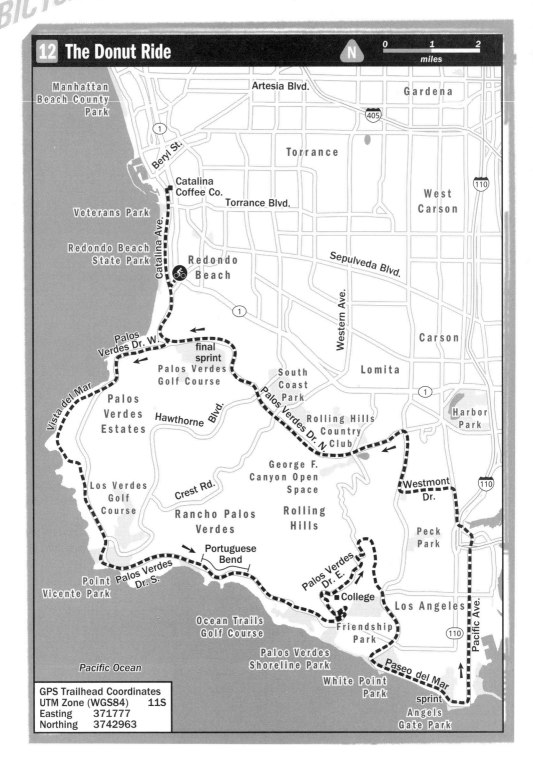

12 The Donut Ride

N

0   1   2
miles

Manhattan
Beach County
Park

Artesia Blvd.

Gardena

405

1

Beryl St.

Catalina
Coffee Co.

Torrance Blvd.

Torrance

West
Carson

110

Veterans Park

Redondo Beach
State Park

Sepulveda Blvd.

Redondo
Beach

Catalina Ave.

1

Carson

Palos
Verdes Dr. W.

final
sprint

Palos Verdes
Golf Course

South
Coast
Park

Lomita

Vista del Mar

Palos
Verdes
Estates

Hawthorne Blvd.

Palos Verdes Dr. N.

Rolling Hills
Country
Club

Western Ave.

1

Harbor
Park

Los Verdes
Golf Course

Crest Rd.

George F.
Canyon Open
Space

Rancho Palos
Verdes

Rolling
Hills

Westmont
Dr.

110

Point
Vicente Park

Palos Verdes
Dr. S.

Portuguese
Bend

Palos Verdes
Dr. E.

College

Peck
Park

Los Angeles

Pacific Ave.

Ocean Trails
Golf Course

Friendship
Park

110

Pacific Ocean

Palos Verdes
Shoreline Park

White Point
Park

Paseo del Mar

sprint

Angels
Gate Park

GPS Trailhead Coordinates
UTM Zone (WGS84)   11S
Easting   371777
Northing   3742963

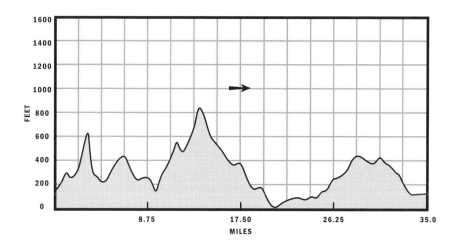

The ride heads south on South Elena Avenue for one block and turns left on South Catalina Avenue. One block later, Catalina intersects Palos Verdes Boulevard, where the group turns right and rises gently to the Palos Verdes Estates town line. The pavement isn't the best here; keep an eye out for potholes. The road quickly dips around a right bend and rises to the Malaga Cove shopping center; the road's name changes to Palos Verdes Drive West at the bend. The center features Italian-inspired architecture and a beautiful fountain in the middle of the parking lot, but you aren't likely to have time to look around if you're with the group.

Palos Verdes Drive West has a wide shoulder to the right, but parked cars frequently force the group into the traffic lane. Whether alone or with the group, do what you can to stay to the right. The road sheds a little elevation for the next half-mile—the group coasts through here—and the road bends just enough to prevent you from seeing too far up ahead. The next mile climbs 260 feet, and it's a great indicator of just how frisky the group is feeling.

After topping out above Bluff Cove, the ride turns right on Paseo Del Mar. The turn is narrow, and coming out of it riders accelerate into the 1.5-mile descent. The road is very wide here and passes through a strictly residential area; traffic is almost nonexistent. The runout is short-lived, and the group turns on the gas for the rise to the right turn on Via Anacapa. Two blocks on, turn right on Via Pacheco for the final kick up to the right turn back onto Palos Verdes Drive West. Almost immediately after your turn, Palos Verdes Drive West becomes Palos Verdes Drive South; you'll notice no difference.

Once on Palos Verdes Drive South, the group will accelerate yet again. Approaching Point Vicente, the road dips and then bends to the right for a little power hill that the group sprints over. The hill is immediately followed by another dip to give you a chance to catch your breath, and that leads into a longer, though shallower, hill. On your own, this rise is no big deal; with the group, many riders are put in trouble. If you have been riding at or near the back, be careful; this is a spot where a few riders always seem to get dropped. Over the top is another downhill; this one is quick but straight. Rounding Abalone Point, the road narrows from two lanes to one and the shoulder is very narrow. The group will slow for the next rise, in part because Botts' dots cover the width of the lane. It's easy to pass between rows of them, but even if you hit the dots, they are small enough to ride over. This field of Botts' dots signals the beginning of Portuguese Bend.

The road through Portuguese Bend is a mile-long stretch of asphalt built on top of land that is perpetually in motion. It undulates and bumps like a salsa dancer, though with considerably less rhythm. Stay in the drops and keep your weight centered over the bike, and you'll sail through this section with only a few pedal strokes. After passing through a notch cut into the hillside, you'll be back on solid ground.

Let's hope you're feeling good because you are at the foot of the day's biggest challenge. The next 3 miles climb 700 feet at an average gradient of only 4.5 percent. Thanks to a few flat spots, the steep sections are more like 7 percent. There is a shoulder here, but it is not terribly wide, and, with a median dividing the two traffic lanes, staying right and out of the way of traffic requires a bit of effort.

Move into the left lane and turn onto Palos Verdes Drive East. The next 2 miles up are what locals call "the switchbacks"— arguably the hardest part of the whole ride. At the top, turn right into the parking lot of Marymount School. This is a great opportunity to recover; the group will stay here for a few minutes while slower riders arrive.

The route continues on Palos Verdes Drive East. The ensuing descent will give you a chance to spin your legs a bit as you cruise through the next few bends. Turn right at Miraleste Plaza and immediately right again on Miraleste Drive. The next 1.25 miles descend much more quickly but flatten out before the next turn. The group turns right at Western Avenue. Be careful in the turn; there is frequently some loose

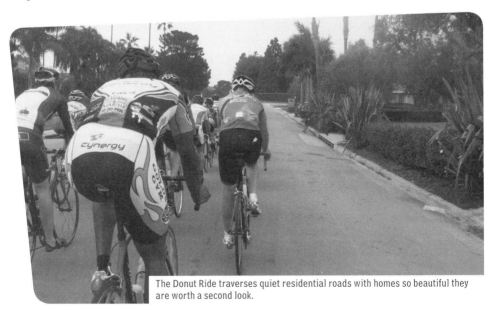

The Donut Ride traverses quiet residential roads with homes so beautiful they are worth a second look.

gravel. Following two short hills, Western crosses West 25th Street and begins the fastest descent of the ride. Provided there is no headwind coming off the ocean, speeds upward of 45 mph are possible. The descent ends with a left bend into West Paseo Del Mar; the group will take the turn single file without braking.

The next 1.7 miles constitute the single flattest stretch of the ride. It culminates in a sprint just before Point Fermin. Coast on by the lighthouse at Point Fermin; West Paseo Del Mar becomes Shepard Street. Turn left at South Pacific Avenue. The group will soft pedal here to give everyone a chance to recover. There is a bike lane, though traffic is light if you departed early. Following a brief downhill that bends left, move into the left lane, turn onto West Channel Street, pass under I-110, and immediately turn right on North Gaffey Street. The next half-mile is mercifully flat, but this will be the end of the peace.

The group will move into the left lane and turn onto Westmont Drive. The group rides this 1-mile climb at a firm tempo but backs off for the right turn onto Western Avenue. A quick downhill runs into yet another rise that precedes the left turn onto Palos Verdes Drive North. There is an alternate finish to the ride, called the Post Loop. It adds another 13 miles and 1,200 feet of climbing to the route.

The next 5 miles can be pretty brutal. There are three distinct hills. The first follows the intersection with Palos Verdes Drive North, the second comes after you cross Crenshaw Boulevard, and the final follows Hawthorne Boulevard. The only opportunities to recover occur if the group is stopped by one of the four lights on Palos Verdes Drive North.

Following the stop sign at Via Opata, the group makes a final acceleration and sprint. Though there's no line for the sprint,

The Donut Ride is an institution in South Bay cycling culture. The ride dates to 1973 and has maintained a reputation for being both beautiful and challenging.

it finishes roughly 1.1 miles from Via Opata. The finish is quick because it unfolds on a downhill. Immediately afterward, make the dogleg right turn onto Via Capay. Set up to the left for the chicane at the bottom of the hill, and you'll cruise through with no brakes. At the top of the rise, follow your recovering compatriots left onto Via Anita and around the downhill left bend. Turn right on Palos Verdes Boulevard and follow the downhill to the left onto Catalina Avenue. The final, flat 2 miles will be a relaxed ride to the coffee shop.

The Post-Loop: Generally, a small group of riders will climb Palos Verdes Drive East a second time. On the approach to Palos Verdes Drive East, watch for riders to begin splitting off from the group; move with them to the left lane and wait for the turn arrow. This ascent of the north side of the hill takes in the highest point on this side, Crest Drive and the radar domes. The climb is 6 miles and gains more than 1,200 feet of elevation in that span for an average gradient of only 4 percent.

With a reasonably wide shoulder, a slower pace than earlier, and a small group, the climb isn't too frenetic. Just past Rockinghorse Road, the road eases into a short descent into the neighborhood of Miraleste. The big-ring cruise will feel good after the sustained climb. But the free ride ends quickly, and, following a bend to the right, you get a reminder of just how rough things can be, with a short stretch at 9 percent. The ongoing changes in pitch mean it is important that you stay in a small gear so you can accelerate when the grade permits.

Turn right at Crest Road. The road turns up steeply, but this short 12-percent grade is the worst you'll experience on the ride. The challenge is to get back on top of the gear when the grade backs down to a more manageable 8 percent. You'll encounter a brief flat 0.7 miles from the top, but the final push to the top will present no surprises. Take a moment to have a bite to eat before descending to the coast.

Turn right at Palos Verdes Drive East and follow the switchbacks to Palos Verdes Drive South. Though you traveled this road only an hour earlier, it will seem utterly fresh to you in this direction. The wide shoulder will put some space between you and the traffic that has picked up since you were first here. Passing into Portuguese Bend, it would be wise to move into the traffic lane a bit because the closer to the edge you are, the more the asphalt tends to undulate; some of the bumps have been known to eject bottles from their cages.

With more than 2 hours of hills in your legs, you are likely to be feeling a little tired, so the hills at Abalone Cove and Point Vicente will be tough. Fortunately, there's only one more serious hill to go.

Turn right on Via Montemar; the road will intersect Via Del Monte. Turn left and follow Via Del Monte downhill. Turn left at Via Chico and pass downhill through the brick arch, then immediately turn right onto Palos Verdes Drive West. Once there, move into the left lane and follow the road through a left-hand dip, and then move to the shoulder on the right. At the top of the rise, move into the left turn lane and turn left onto Paseo de la Playa. The road will bend to the right and descend toward the beach. At Esplanade, turn left; there is a bike lane here, and you get a great view of the ocean. At Knob Hill, turn right and immediately turn left on Catalina Avenue to follow the others to the coffee shop.

After the Ride
Many riders will stop at a locally owned coffee shop in Redondo Beach following the ride. Catalina Coffee Co. is known for having great coffee and a diverse menu, and for being the unofficial end point for all rides in the South Bay. If you're looking for burgers and fries, Mexican food, or seafood, try the restaurants in Hollywood Riviera, where the ride started.

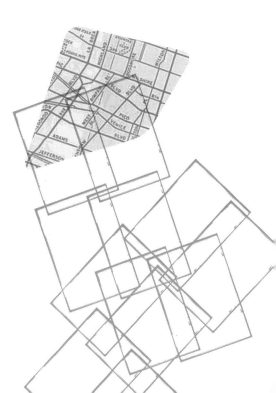

13 Palos Verdes Estates Loop

AT A GLANCE

Length: 12.4 miles

Configuration: Loop

Difficulty: Moderate

Climbing: 1,300 feet

Maximum gradient: 11%

Scenery: Mountains, ocean, an island, and immaculately manicured lawns

Exposure: Mornings are frequently overcast

Road traffic: Light, except for Palos Verdes Boulevard

Road surface: Good, except in Portuguese Bend

Riding time: 90 minutes, with stops

Maps: Los Angeles County *Thomas Guide* pages 792, 793, and 822

In Brief

This is a very scenic ride that takes riders up a climb onto the Palos Verdes Peninsula. Overlooks on the climb will offer million-dollar views of the Angeles Crest and Santa Monica Mountains and Catalina Island.

Directions

This ride begins in south Redondo Beach in a neighborhood known as Hollywood Riviera. To get there, exit I-405 at Hawthorne Boulevard, southbound. Hawthorne intersects I-405 south of Los Angeles International Airport and I-105 and west of I-110. You'll drive south on Hawthorne 5.2 miles, until you reach the Pacific Coast Highway (PCH). There, turn right and drive 1.4 miles to Avenue I, where you will turn left. Immediately turn left onto South Elena Avenue. At the southwest corner of South Elena Avenue and Avenida Del Norte is a large, metered parking lot. If you prefer free parking, you can usually find some on one of the neighborhood's side streets.

Description

This ride is largely without flat; the road will generally be going either up or down, which is why a ride of this length gets a moderate difficulty rating. Your efforts will be rewarded with some of the most commanding views available in the South Bay. One note: There are many stop signs on this ride. Police in both Redondo Beach and Palos Verdes Estates are inclined to ticket cyclists who roll through stop signs, and the tickets are not cheap.

To begin the ride, exit the parking lot at the west side onto Vista Del Mar. Travel southwest on Vista Del Mar to Esplanade, where you turn left. You'll get a glimpse of the ocean view that you'll see much more of as the ride progresses. Esplanade becomes Calle Miramar, and the road climbs uphill gently. Following a left-hand bend, turn right onto Camino de Encanto. The road flattens briefly before resuming its climb up to Paseo de la Playa, at which point

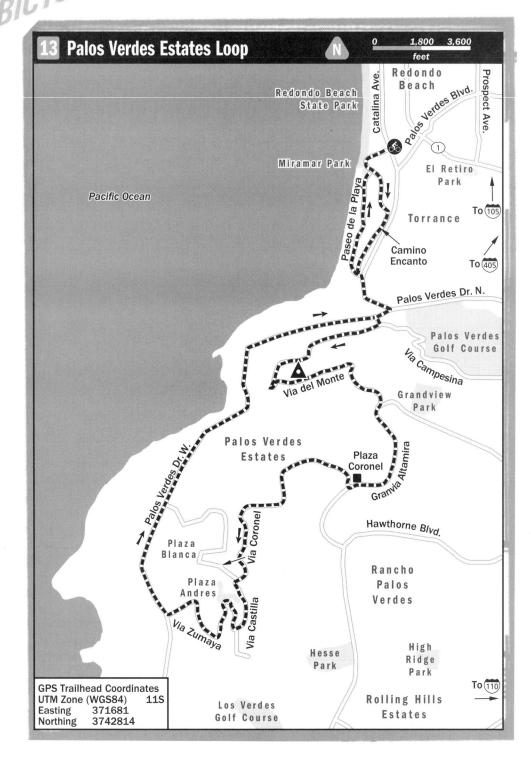

13 Palos Verdes Estates Loop

N

0   1,800   3,600
feet

Redondo Beach
State Park

Redondo Beach

Catalina Ave.

Palos Verdes Blvd.

Prospect Ave.

Miramar Park

El Retiro Park

1

To 105

Paseo de la Playa

Torrance

Pacific Ocean

Camino Encanto

To 405

Palos Verdes Dr. N.

Palos Verdes Golf Course

Via Campesina

Via del Monte

Grandview Park

Palos Verdes Estates

Plaza Coronel

Granvia Altamira

Palos Verdes Dr. W.

Hawthorne Blvd.

Plaza Blanca

Via Coronel

Rancho Palos Verdes

Plaza Andres

Via Castilla

Via Zumaya

High Ridge Park

Hesse Park

Los Verdes Golf Course

To 110

Rolling Hills Estates

GPS Trailhead Coordinates
UTM Zone (WGS84)   11S
Easting   371681
Northing   3742814

BICYCLING

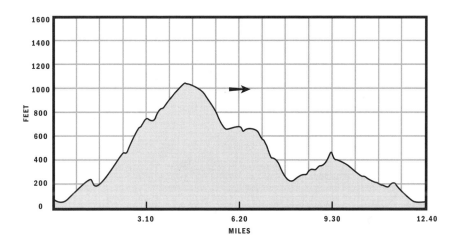

the climb ends and you turn left and then immediately turn right onto Palos Verdes Boulevard. You'll notice an immediate change in the foliage, thanks to an incredible density of trees. The road narrows to a single lane and dips before curling to the right and demanding a small kick up a rise to your next turn. Watch the traffic to your left—traffic from another street is introduced as a second lane. At the top of the rise, move across the second lane and into the turn lane, and then turn into the parking lot of the Malaga Cove shopping center.

The cluster of shops features striking Mediterranean architecture and is accented by a beautiful fountain at its center. You'll notice a high archway as you make your turn. Pass under the archway and spin up the slight rise to Via Del Monte, where you turn right. You'll have a short (100-yard) flat before the big attraction of this ride starts. The climb up Via Del Monte and on to the terminus of the ascent is roughly 3 miles, with a significant flat about midway up the climb.

Palos Verdes Estates is one of the most affluent communities in Los Angeles County—and it shows. The homes here are unfailingly gorgeous, with architectural features to capitalize on their truly million-dollar views. And because beautiful homes demand equally beautiful lawns, you'll see an incredible array of flora. The area's mild climate means you'll see three or four varieties of lavender, plus hydrangea, California poppy, bougainvillea, bird of paradise, many different roses, and more. This is one climb worth taking it easy on and looking around.

Via Del Monte is a lightly traveled residential street and features a wide shoulder for much of the climb. Your best views initially will be on your right. Between a few of the homes, you'll be able to see the beach extending from Torrance through Redondo and Hermosa beaches up to Manhattan Beach. On clear days, you'll be able to see across the bay to the Santa Monica Mountains in Malibu.

Shortly after the climb's only switchback, the gradient gently rolls off to a flat approximately 200 yards long. The north side of the street features a steep hillside and is devoid of homes; this is the perfect spot to pull over and take in one of the best views in the area. To the northeast, you'll see the San Gabriel Mountains; to northwest, you'll take in a much better view of the Santa Monica Mountains and the coastline of Malibu clear to Point Dume.

These places give new meaning to the term "trophy home." Take the descent with a bit of caution: some of the pitches on this side reach grades of 13 percent. The route down will be very twisty and requires your full attention. You'll pass Via Fernandez and, following a left-hand bend, will hit a rise that's likely to be just a little too long

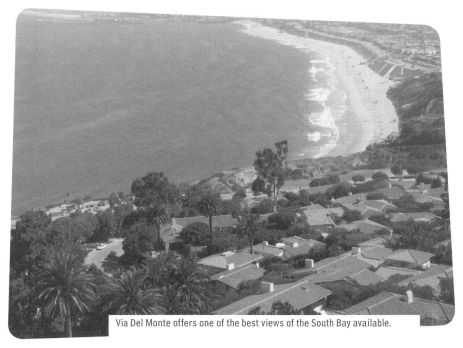

Via Del Monte offers one of the best views of the South Bay available.

At this point, you have completed roughly half the climb. Remount your bike and continue on Via Del Monte. The road quickly turns to its steepest grade as you exit a right-hand bend. Fortunately, the grade tips up to 11 percent only briefly. When you reach the T-intersection with Granvia Altamira, turn right. The climb will continue on this road until you reach Plaza Coronel, a sizable grass plot.

On the other side of Plaza Coronel, you will begin your descent back to the coast. As if the architecture could get any more impressive, you'll pass some homes worthy of your slowing down to take a gander.

for you to power through. Once the road turns down again, it bends to the right and you turn left onto Via Castillo. You'll take in another brief rise before the road turns down for the final section of descent.

Turn right onto Via Zumaya. You'll encounter a rise short enough to take in your big ring before the asphalt peels away from you rather steeply. This can be a rollicking fun descent with its many turns, but it's probably a good idea to be conservative if this is your first time down this road. At the stop sign at Palos Verdes Drive West, turn right. There is a wide shoulder here, but parked cars can force you into the traffic lane briefly; conditions are usually quiet, so you should be able to hear if any cars are approaching from behind.

Palos Verdes is known for its cliffs that overlook the coves so popular with divers and surfers. After passing through the neighborhood of Lunada Bay, you encounter a dramatic view of these cliffs to your left. There is even a parking area, should you wish to stop for a photo or two—it's truly a special view. Next, the road will climb once more and bend around one of the highest of the cliffs. Your effort will be rewarded by an easy descent back to Malaga Cove. And though the road has a few bends to it, you should be able to tackle this without hitting your brakes. This is one of the most traveled roads on the Palos Verdes Peninsula, so be aware of traffic approaching from behind you. If there's no traffic present, though, it is safest to take the whole of the lane for the descent.

As you approach Malaga Cove, the road will turn upward once again, but this rise will be both shallow and brief. The shopping center is the one you passed earlier in the ride. When the road divides into two lanes, move into the left lane to take Palos Verdes Boulevard back into Redondo Beach and to your vehicle. The three-way intersection of Palos Verdes Boulevard, Palos Verdes Boulevard North, and Palos Verdes Boulevard West (what you are on) has the potential to be hazardous for cyclists because each approach to the intersection is downhill, and drivers can misjudge your speed. After passing through the intersection, quickly move to the right lane and on into the bike lane.

Approximately 200 yards after the intersection, you will reach the left turn back onto Paseo de la Playa. Traffic approaching from the rear is likely to be traveling fast, so be extra careful as you cross the two lanes of traffic to the turn lane. After turning left

onto Paseo de la Playa, take it directly back to Esplanade; you'll get one final ocean view before the end of the ride. At Esplanade, turn left and then turn right immediately afterward onto Vista Del Mar, which will deliver you back to the parking lot.

After the Ride

Exiting the parking lot, you are within walking distance of coffee shops and a variety of restaurants. From American fare to Mexican and French-style baked goods, you have many choices within 100 yards.

Your efforts will be rewarded with some of the most commanding views available in the South Bay.

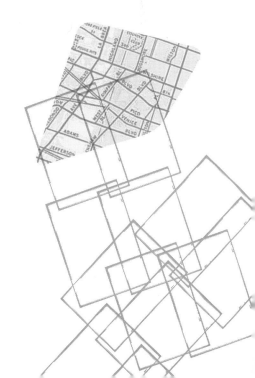

14 The Pier Ride

AT A GLANCE

Length: 28 miles

Configuration: Loop

Difficulty: Moderate (solo), difficult (group)

Climbing: 400 feet

Maximum gradient: 6%

Scenery: Beach, ocean, the boats of Marina Del Rey, and Los Angeles International Airport

Exposure: Mornings are frequently overcast

Road traffic: Moderate, except for Pershing Avenue, which can be heavy

Road surface: Good

Riding time: 2 hours

Maps: Los Angeles County *Thomas Guide* pages 732, 702, 701, 672, and 671

In Brief

Marina Del Rey is LA's largest marina for private boat owners. This loop takes riders up the bike path from Manhattan Beach, through the marina, and up to a road that parallels the airport, giving cyclists an excellent view of the planes taking off and landing at one of the world's busiest airports.

Directions

Manhattan Beach is the starting point for this ride.

From I-405 southbound: Exit at Inglewood Avenue, turn right, and stay in the right lane. Turn right onto Manhattan Beach Boulevard and drive west 3 miles toward the beach. Metered parking in Manhattan Beach is plentiful, and there is a parking garage just north of Manhattan Beach Boulevard that can be reached by turning right on Morningside Drive. There is limited parking at the pier, so you'd best look for parking on the eastern edge of downtown.

From I-405 northbound: Exit at Hawthorne Boulevard and turn right. Immediately move into the left lane to turn onto Manhattan Beach Boulevard, then travel west (toward the beach) 3.3 miles and follow the directions above for parking.

Description

Finding flat roads in Los Angeles where you can have a good hard ride without worrying too much about traffic can be, well, difficult. This circuit gives you a few opportunities to drill it into the red zone without much fear of traffic or terrorizing others on the bike path. The ride is generally flat, with only a few modest rises. On Tuesdays and Thursdays, you can join a group that does this ride year-round. The group meets at 6:30 a.m. at the Manhattan Beach Pier.

Roll out north on the beach bike path. In El Porto, north of Rosecrans Avenue, you will need to watch for surfers heading out to catch the morning waves. The group

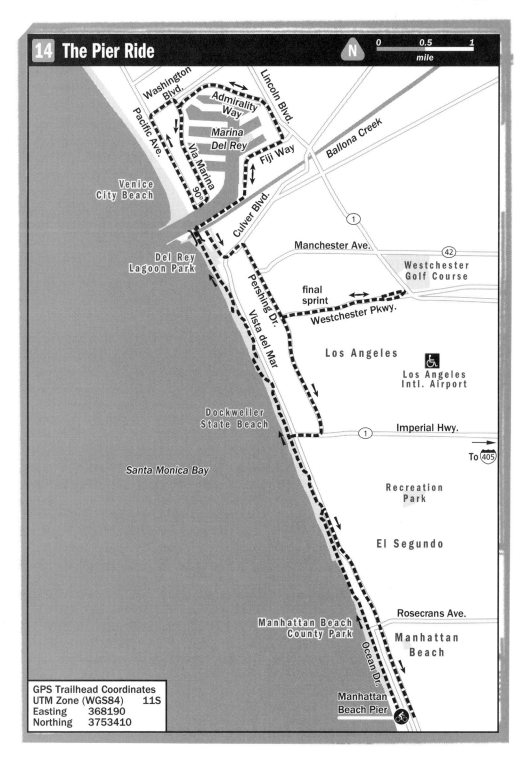

14 **The Pier Ride**

N

0   0.5   1
mile

Washington Blvd.

Lincoln Blvd.

Admirality Way

Pacific Ave.

Marina Del Rey

Via Marina

Fiji Way

Ballona Creek

90°

Venice City Beach

Culver Blvd.

1

Manchester Ave.

42

Del Rey Lagoon Park

Westchester Golf Course

final sprint

Pershing Dr.

Westchester Pkwy.

Los Angeles

Los Angeles Intl. Airport

Vista del Mar

Dockweiler State Beach

Imperial Hwy.

1

To 405

Santa Monica Bay

Recreation Park

El Segundo

Rosecrans Ave.

Manhattan Beach County Park

Manhattan Beach

Ocean Dr.

Manhattan Beach Pier

GPS Trailhead Coordinates
UTM Zone (WGS84)   11S
Easting   368190
Northing   3753410

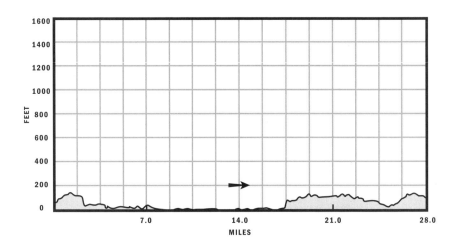

pedals at an easy pace up the path and rides in a double-file paceline. This early in the morning, the temperature is generally cool, except in July and August.

The ride will cross the bridge in Playa Del Rey and continue up the jetty. The group ride will pick up a few more riders waiting at the bridge. Follow the path's left turn to Fiji Way and exit the bike path. Fiji Way turns right just beyond a collection of restaurants and tourist shops called Fisherman's Village. Traffic here is very light for three reasons: 1) Fiji dead-ends at the bike path; 2) Fiji is bordered to the south by the Ballona Creek Wetlands, an area that is fenced off; and 3) the businesses here are boat retailers and restaurants, and they don't open until at least 10 a.m.

Turn left at Admiralty Way. The group ride will just begin to pick up the pace. Following the left turn, quickly get into the right lane. There are lights at Mindanao Way and Bali Way that usually interrupt riders' acceleration, but after that you are usually rewarded with a straight shot all the way to Via Marina, your next turn. In season, the group ride will frequently accelerate up to 30 mph, but during the winter the speed may rise no higher than 25 or 26 mph. Also, if you choose to do the group rides, it is helpful to know that Thursday's ride tends to be just a little slower than Tuesday's is.

If you're riding on your own, this is a great opportunity to look out onto the water and view ships entering and leaving the marina via the channel; you can also view the jetty you recently rode down.

Turn left at Via Marina; this begins a 2.2-mile loop that will be largely devoid of traffic. Via Marina bends right; 300 yards farther, make a sharp right turn onto Pacific Avenue for the mile-long run to Washington Boulevard. (Traffic and a new stop sign ended the sprint.)

Ease up and coast to the light at Washington Boulevard. Turn right and ride 0.3 miles to Via Marina, then turn right. The group will go a little slower here, but they won't soft pedal. Make sure you stay tucked in. Following the right turn, immediately move to the left lane to turn back onto Admiralty Way.

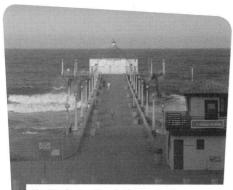

The Manhattan Beach Pier is a local landmark and the start point of the weekday morning group ride the Pier Ride.

As you turn onto Admiralty, watch for cars turning right onto Admiralty from northbound Via Marina. A right-turn lane guides traffic into the right lane without having it stop. Riders must pause to check for cars entering before moving into the right lane. Even seeing a large group, some drivers will accelerate to outrun it. Once the group has moved into the right lane, it will begin to accelerate. On your right is the marina itself, and in between several restaurants and hotels you get great views of basins C and D, that is, if you're on your own. In the group, you won't be looking around much; you'll be responding to the group's acceleration here and working to stay tucked in.

As you round the bend bringing you to Bali Way, watch for the light; it comes up suddenly. The route continues to double back on Admiralty; turn right at Fiji Way. Because this is a T-intersection with a right-turn arrow, you won't have to stop before turning. The group sprints out of the turn and makes a mammoth acceleration before reaching the loop that leads you back onto the bike path. Make sure to stay right to allow room for riders exiting the bike path as you ride up the ramp.

Bear right to head west on the jetty. Early in the day there is little offshore wind, but in the afternoon it begins picking up. By late afternoon, it's a steady blow that feels like the brakes are rubbing. The group slows down here; the jetty isn't terribly wide. Turn left onto the bridge and get ready for an unusual transition.

There is a guardrail that designates the end of Pacific Avenue, separating it from the bridge. Ride down off the curb and south on Pacific. The group will break into two pacelines here—both to the right of the guardrail but separated by a pole. Just 200 meters down Pacific, turn left on Convoy Street. You will follow this with an immediate right onto Esplanade and a left onto Culver Boulevard. Though traffic here is light, watch for cars on Culver before crossing it. The light at the intersection of Culver and Vista Del Mar is rarely green when you nose up to the intersection, but don't worry—the recovery couldn't hurt.

Immediately after crossing Vista Del Mar, bear right onto Pershing Drive. You will climb 50 feet in the next 0.4 miles. It's not a lot, but after a dead-flat ride so far it can feel like a mountain, especially if you hit it at more than 20 mph. Pershing curves to the right as it climbs; another half-mile after the road flattens, move to the left lane.

Turn left on Westchester Parkway. This 2.3-mile stretch of road is LA's answer to the drag strip . . . for bicycles. It is almost entirely straight and features less than 300 feet of elevation gain—including the return trip.

There is a wide shoulder and bike lane here. Even if you're alone and cars pass you at 55 or 60 mph, you have enough room between you and them to keep you feeling safe. The group rides double file here, though there are usually a few riders who will venture into the traffic lane.

To your right, you will see Los Angeles International Airport. Your view is an unusually unobstructed one of the planes on the runways and taxiways. This is a rare opportunity to see the workings of one of the world's busiest airports. The group hammers through this stretch; sometimes the pace is high enough to reduce the bunch to single-file suffering.

Just beyond the intersection with La Tijera Boulevard, a central median comes to an end. The group makes a U-turn here, clear of the crush of traffic. Thanks to the median, the U-turn can be made in two parts; move to the middle first, and once you can see there is no oncoming traffic finish the turn. The final stretch of the ride is your opportunity to see what your legs have left in them. The group keeps its pace high in anticipation of a final sprint roughly 100 yards before the intersection with Falmouth Avenue.

When you return to Pershing Drive, turn left. Here the group begins to break up; riders who live in the South Bay will continue south 1.5 miles on Pershing, whereas those who live on the west side will head north.

Turn right at Imperial Highway and ride 0.3 miles to Vista Del Mar. Turn left and ride 3.5 miles south to Highland Avenue. If you are alone, you may wish to go straight and follow the driveway down to the beach bike path. The group stays on the road for a quicker return to Manhattan Beach.

After the Ride
Many riders stop for coffee in town following the ride. Downtown Manhattan Beach has a variety of shops, stores, cafes, and restaurants to choose from. One needn't stray far from the central drag to find a great opportunity to refuel.

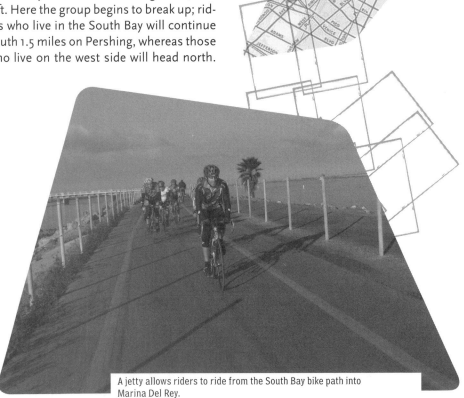

A jetty allows riders to ride from the South Bay bike path into Marina Del Rey.

15 Palos Verdes Estates Golf Course Loop

AT A GLANCE

Length: 6 miles
Configuration: Loop
Difficulty: Easy
Climbing: 300 feet

Maximum gradient: 6%

Scenery: Ocean and one of the prettiest golf courses in Los Angeles County

Exposure: Mornings are frequently overcast

Road traffic: Light, except for Palos Verdes Boulevard

Road surface: Good

Riding time: 30 minutes

Maps: Los Angeles County *Thomas Guide* pages 792 and 793

In Brief

This easy route takes riders out of Redondo Beach and into the idyllic seclusion of the Palos Verdes Peninsula. By focusing on the northern side of the peninsula, riders take advantage of shallower grades with a gentle rise. The views around the golf course are a peaceful oasis in LA's sprawling metropolis.

Directions

This ride begins in south Redondo Beach in a neighborhood known as Hollywood Riviera. To get there, exit I-405 at Hawthorne Boulevard southbound. Hawthorne intersects I-405 south of Los Angeles International Airport and I-105 and west of I-110. Drive south on Hawthorne 5.2 miles, until you reach the Pacific Coast Highway (PCH), where you will turn right, drive 1.4 miles, then turn left onto Avenue I. Make an immediate left turn onto South Elena Avenue. At the southwest corner of South

Elena Avenue and Avenida Del Norte is a large, metered parking lot. If you prefer free parking, you can usually find some on one of the neighborhood's side streets.

Description

This ride is almost never flat and, as a result, your views are ever-changing as you pedal along. The grades are gentle enough that this ride can be done on almost any sort of bike, including a beach cruiser, though hills are always easier with low gears. Restrooms can be found at the coffee shops and the gas station, or along the beach below Esplanade.

One note: There are many stop signs on this ride. Police in both Redondo Beach and Palos Verdes Estates are inclined to ticket cyclists who roll through them, and the tickets are not cheap.

To begin the ride, pedal southwest out of the parking lot on Vista Del Mar. At Esplanade, turn left; you will spy the beach

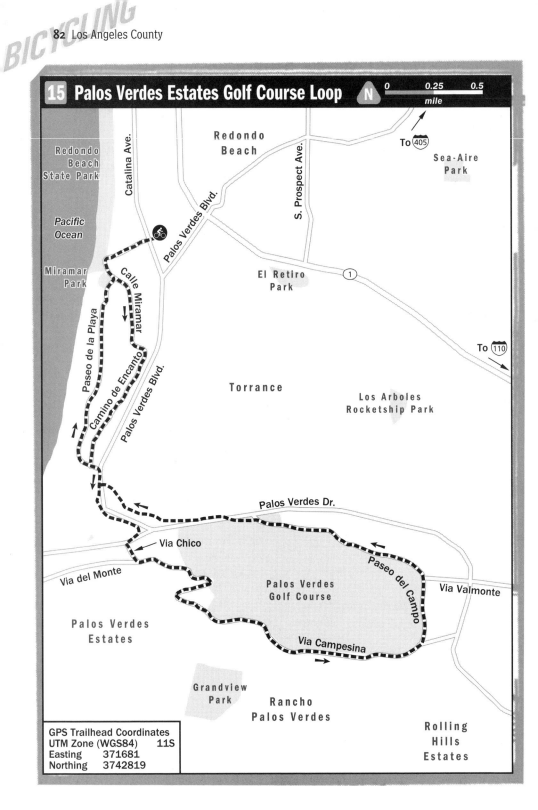

15 Palos Verdes Estates Golf Course Loop

N

0   0.25   0.5
mile

Redondo
Beach

To 405

Sea-Aire
Park

Redondo
Beach
State Park

Catalina Ave.

S. Prospect Ave.

Palos Verdes Blvd.

Pacific
Ocean

Miramar
Park

Calle Miramar

El Retiro
Park

1

To 110

Paseo de la Playa

Camino de Encanto

Palos Verdes Blvd.

Torrance

Los Arboles
Rocketship Park

Palos Verdes Dr.

Via Chico

Via del Monte

Palos Verdes
Golf Course

Paseo del Campo

Via Valmonte

Palos Verdes
Estates

Via Campesina

Grandview
Park

Rancho
Palos Verdes

Rolling
Hills
Estates

GPS Trailhead Coordinates
UTM Zone (WGS84)   11S
Easting   371681
Northing   3742819

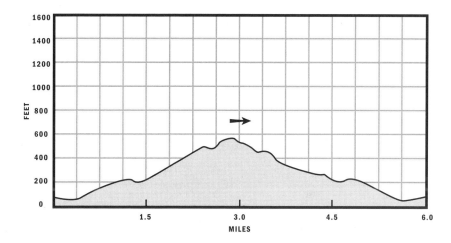

below and the cliffs of the Palos Verdes Peninsula. Esplanade becomes Calle Miramar as it begins a gentle climb toward Palos Verdes. At Camino de Encanto, turn right and continue through the residential neighborhood. At the top of the hill, you will reach Paseo de la Playa. Turn left and then immediately turn right onto Palos Verdes Boulevard. This road has a sizable shoulder initially, but it narrows at the bottom of the dip where Palos Verdes Boulevard meets Palos Verdes Boulevard North; take the lane and make a short effort up to your next turn at Via Chico in Malaga Cove Plaza.

One of the remarkable aspects of Palos Verdes Estates is how different the foliage is relative to the rest of the South Bay. Upon entering the community, you will notice a preponderance of eucalyptus trees. For many, the area reminds them of the Monterey Peninsula. Unlike some areas in the greater Los Angeles basin, trees here are plentiful and varied. In addition to eucalyptus, you'll see cypress, oak, and various evergreens. The incredible affluence of the residents can, of course, be seen in the architecture of the homes, but the landscaping can be opulent enough to draw attention away from the dwellings themselves. Lovers of annuals will see hydrangea, lily of the valley, lavender, poppy, nasturtium, and more variations on the rose than you'll see in some nurseries.

You will see the plaza on your left, but Via Chico will not be signed. However, you will know it by the large brick archway at the north end of the plaza. Ride under the archway and up the brief hill, then turn left on Via Campesina.

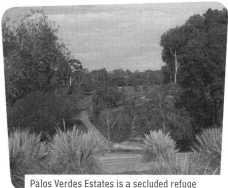

Palos Verdes Estates is a secluded refuge from bustling Los Angeles.

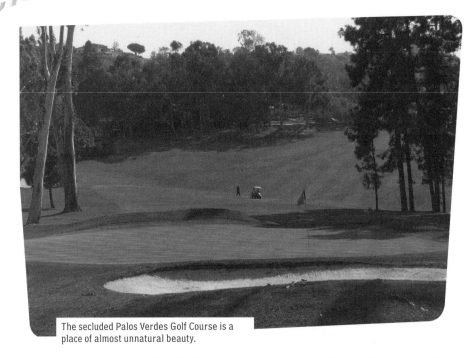

The secluded Palos Verdes Golf Course is a place of almost unnatural beauty.

Via Campesina twists and bends for the next 1.3 miles on its way to Palos Verdes Country Club. The road here climbs steadily uphill, but there are some dips to break up the climb and make the ride more enjoyable. The rise concludes just beyond Yellow Brick Road (seriously). To your left is the Emerald City (just kidding). Pull over anywhere along the top of this rise for a truly spectacular view, then continue on Via Campesina, heading downhill now. Turn left at Paseo Del Campo, where you will continue to hug the edge of the golf course on a gentle downhill run. Watch for the speed bumps intended to keep SUVs from setting local land-speed records.

Paseo Del Campo intersects Palos Verdes Drive North and becomes Via Alameda. Cross Palos Verdes Drive North to Via Alameda and immediately turn left onto Via Capay. The road will run downhill to a right–left chicane that turns very sharply; brake in advance and then get back on the gas for the short run up to the left turn onto Via Anita. This road will head back downhill and bend left before ending at Palos Verdes Boulevard.

Turn right onto Palos Verdes Boulevard and get into the left lane immediately to turn back onto Paseo de la Playa. Traffic approaching from the rear is likely to be traveling fast, so be extra careful as you cross the two lanes of traffic to the turn lane. After turning onto Paseo de la Playa, take it directly back to Esplanade; you'll get one final ocean view before the end of the ride. At Esplanade, turn left, and then immediately turn right onto Vista Del Mar, which delivers you back to the parking lot.

After the Ride
Exiting the parking lot, you are within walking distance of coffee shops and a variety of restaurants. From American fare to Mexican and French-style baked goods, you have many choices within 100 yards.

16 The Radar Domes

AT A GLANCE	**Length:** 33 miles
	Configuration: Loop
	Difficulty: Difficult
	Climbing: 5,200 feet

Maximum gradient: 13%

Scenery: Ocean, Catalina Island, the ports of San Pedro and Long Beach, and the Santa Monica and San Gabriel mountains

Exposure: Mornings are frequently overcast

Road traffic: Light, except for Palos Verdes Boulevard North

Road surface: Good, except for Portuguese Bend

Riding time: 2.5 hours

Maps: Los Angeles County *Thomas Guide* pages 792, 793, 823, and 822

In Brief

This challenging loop takes riders out of Redondo Beach and onto the many climbs of the Palos Verdes Peninsula, offering a selection of great ascents followed by some very fun descents. And you'll definitely see why people say the homes here have million-dollar views.

Directions

This ride begins in south Redondo Beach in a neighborhood known as Hollywood Riviera. To get there, exit I-405 at Hawthorne Boulevard southbound. Hawthorne intersects I-405 south of Los Angeles International Airport and I-105 and west of I-110. Drive south on Hawthorne 5.2 miles, until you reach the Pacific Coast Highway (PCH), where you will turn right. Drive 1.4 miles and turn left onto Avenue I. Immediately turn left again onto South Elena Avenue. At the southwest corner of South Elena Avenue and Avenida Del Norte

is a large, metered parking lot. If you prefer free parking, you can usually find some on one of the neighborhood's side streets.

Description

To begin the ride, exit the parking lot at the west side onto Vista Del Mar. Travel southwest on Vista Del Mar to Esplanade, turn left; you'll catch a glimpse of an ocean view that you'll see more of as the ride progresses. Esplanade becomes Calle Miramar, and the road climbs gently uphill. Following a left-hand bend, turn right onto Camino de Encanto. The road will flatten briefly before resuming its climb up to Paseo de la Playa, where the climb ends, necessitating a turn left and then a quick right turn (less than 50 feet later) onto Palos Verdes Boulevard. You'll notice an immediate change in the foliage, thanks to an incredible density of trees. The road narrows to a single lane, then dips before curling to the right and demanding a small kick up a rise to your

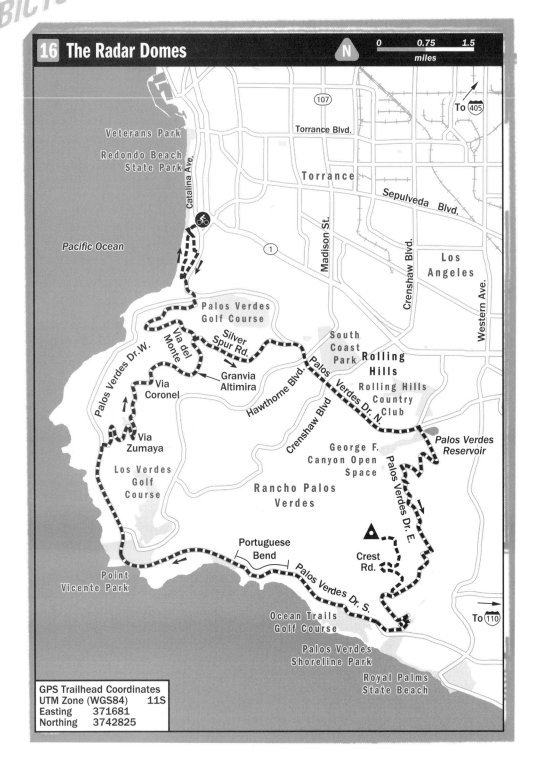

16 The Radar Domes

N

| 0 | 0.75 | 1.5 |

miles

107

To 405

Torrance Blvd.

Veterans Park

Redondo Beach State Park

Torrance

Sepulveda Blvd.

Catalina Ave.

Madison St.

Crenshaw Blvd.

Los Angeles

Western Ave.

Pacific Ocean

1

Palos Verdes Golf Course

Via del Monte

Silver Spur Rd.

South Coast Park

Rolling Hills

Palos Verdes Dr. W.

Via Coronel

Granvia Altimira

Hawthorne Blvd.

Palos Verdes Dr. N.

Rolling Hills Country Club

Palos Verdes Reservoir

Via Zumaya

Los Verdes Golf Course

Crenshaw Blvd

George F. Canyon Open Space

Rancho Palos Verdes

Palos Verdes Dr. E.

Portuguese Bend

Crest Rd.

Point Vicente Park

Palos Verdes Dr. S.

Ocean Trails Golf Course

To 110

Palos Verdes Shoreline Park

Royal Palms State Beach

GPS Trailhead Coordinates
UTM Zone (WGS84)   11S
Easting   371681
Northing   3742825

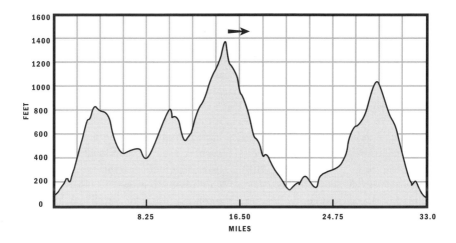

next turn. Watch the traffic to your left as traffic from another street is introduced as a second lane. At the top of the rise, move across the second lane and into the turn lane, and then turn into the parking lot of the Malaga Cove shopping center. Pass through the archway ahead and power up the short hill to Via Del Monte; turn right.

One note: There are many stop signs on this ride. Police in both Redondo Beach and Palos Verdes Estates are inclined to ticket cyclists who roll through them, and the tickets are not cheap.

Palos Verdes Estates is one of the most affluent communities in Los Angeles County—and it shows. The homes here are unfailingly gorgeous, with architectural features to capitalize on their truly million-dollar views. And because beautiful homes demand equally beautiful lawns, you'll see an incredible array of flora. The area's mild climate supports at least four varieties of lavender, plus hydrangea, California poppy, bougainvillea, bird of paradise, a variety of roses, and more. This is one climb worth taking slow to look around.

Via Del Monte is a lightly traveled residential street and features a wide shoulder for much of the climb. On clear days, you'll be able to see across the bay to the Santa Monica Mountains in Malibu.

Shortly after the climb's only switchback, the gradient gently rolls off to a flat that's approximately 200 yards long. The north side of the street features a steep hillside and is devoid of homes; this is the perfect spot to pull over and enjoy one of the best views in the area. To the northeast, look for the San Gabriel Mountains; to the northwest, you'll take in a much better view of the Santa Monica Mountains and the coastline of Malibu clear to Point Dume.

The road quickly turns to its steepest grade as you exit a right-hand bend. Fortunately, the grade tips up to 11 percent only briefly. When you reach the T-intersection with Granvia Altamira, turn left. Granvia Altamira will descend slightly and bend to the right, and the shoulder includes a bike lane. The runout is short to a T-intersection with Silver Spur Lane. Turn left for the descent down Silver Spur.

The road is two lanes with a wide shoulder, but it is wise to take the lane because a cyclist can easily exceed 30 mph on the descent. As you near Palos Verdes Drive North, you will see a right-turn lane with a yield sign. Check for oncoming traffic before merging right onto Palos Verdes Drive North; this is another road with a wide shoulder. You will pass three stoplights—at Hawthorne Boulevard, Crenshaw Boulevard, and Rolling Hills Road—on your way to your next turn. The road will climb slightly on the way to Rolling Hills Road and then gently descend on its way to your next turn.

At Palos Verdes Boulevard East, turn right for the day's biggest climb. This ascent is 7.2 miles long, climbs 1,372 feet, and, thanks to some flat spots, averages just more than a 4-percent gradient. A 1.3-mile-long descent serves to break it up a bit. The first section of the climb wraps through four switchbacks over 2.3 miles and climbs 489 feet with a gradient averaging roughly 4 percent. The descent begins following this section. At Miraleste Road, turn left. You will see a gas station in the shopping center to your right; it has a convenience store, should you need to get a drink. The road will bend to the right and then straighten as it continues to descend. Your next turn will come up rather suddenly. Begin braking when you see the break in the median strip on your left. The intersection is Via Colinita, where you will turn right. Because the turn is downhill and off-camber, it is important to scrub your speed as much as necessary before turning.

Via Colinita is a small residential street with some beautiful homes. It features three distinct switchbacks, and the gradient can vary widely depending on whether you take an inside or outside line; near the top it reaches a maximum gradient of 13 percent. Via Colinita intersects Palos Verdes Drive East; turn left to continue the climb. Following the steep rise to the intersection, you get a brief respite as Palos Verdes Drive East flattens following a right-hand bend. For the next 0.75 miles, the grade will remain fairly gentle. However, that will change.

Turn right on Crest Road. The road immediately kicks up to 12 percent for approximately 60 feet, and though the gradient relaxes some following that, it remains near 8 percent for the next 0.75 miles. Be careful not to make too big an effort on the opening grade or you'll pay dearly. Upon rounding a right-hand switchback, the road goes pancake flat (and smooth), but only for about 100 yards; it's a nice opportunity to recover before the final 0.75-mile push to the top of the climb, which averages 5 percent. At the top, you'll notice a gate blocking further progress, though the road continues. You'll also see the radar dome, a water tank, and an assortment of antennae above you. On clear days, the view to the north includes a wide angle on the Los Angeles basin. You can see downtown, the Hollywood sign and, of course, the curtain that is the San Gabriel Mountains.

Your descent begins when you double back down Crest Road to the intersection with Palos Verdes Drive East. If you need water, cross the intersection to Marymount School and follow the driveway down to the circle; on your left you will see the administration building. Just below a window to the right of the doors of the building is a spigot. Have a bite in the shade of the trees before resuming your descent.

Upon exiting the school's driveway, turn left and descend Palos Verdes Drive East. The winding road offers great views of the ocean, and occasional glimpses of San Pedro, Long Beach, and Catalina Island. The turns on the descent are not difficult; frequently, they are banked, and skilled descenders can maintain speeds above 30 mph to the intersection with Palos Verdes Drive South. Although there is some shoulder here, it is wise to take the whole lane for your descent.

Turn right at Palos Verdes Drive South. There is a wide shoulder here to accommodate cyclists, and it is generally glass-free. To your left is Trump National Golf Course, once the world's only 15-hole course (sinkholes can wreak havoc on careful landscaping), but it is an 18-hole course these days. Continue to descend the next 1.5 miles. The road will bend a bit, but there will be no major turns, and with its gentle grade you'll be able to turn a big gear. It's a really fun section, but be mindful of traffic approaching from behind you—cars can come up on you so quickly they seem to materialize out of thin air.

After passing a wide strip of Botts' dots, you enter Portuguese Bend. The dots are there to alert drivers to the poor condition of the road ahead. Portuguese Bend is just a mile long, and although Caltrans (the California Department of Transportation) can be credited for its unending efforts to keep Palos Verdes Drive South passable, Portuguese Bend is gradually sliding into the ocean. The signs cautioning you to be wary of landslides aren't jokes. This road will undulate unexpectedly and disconcertingly over rolling terrain until you reach a short hill you can pass with a brief out-of-the-saddle effort.

Following the runout from the hill, you will notice a high row of hedges to your right and signs for the Wayfarer's Chapel. This extraordinary structure is a real treasure of Palos Verdes. Designed by Frank Lloyd Wright's son, Lloyd Wright, the structure is largely glass and looks out on pristine gardens and the blue water of the Pacific. Just beyond the driveway, the road will turn up once again for a gradual half-mile slog

up a false flat, part of nearly 4 miles of rolling terrain that will deliver you to your final climb of the day.

Although the climb uses many different streets, it is generally referred to as Via Zumaya because that is the longest, steepest section of the lower half of the climb—grades on Via Zumaya will reach 13 percent. Turn right on Paseo Lunado. It will intersect Via Rivera, where you will turn left and then immediately turn right onto Via Carillo. Turn right onto Via Romero at the next intersection, and then immediately make another right onto Via Zumaya. The next 0.75 miles are the steepest of the day; if ever there was a time to go redline, this is it. The hill will roll off just before your next turn. Have a sip of water.

Turn left at Via Castilla. There is a short hill that flattens out and then descends

This challenging loop takes riders out of Redondo Beach and onto the many climbs of the Palos Verdes Peninsula, offering a selection of great ascents followed by some very fun descents. And you'll definitely see why people say the homes here have million-dollar views.

BICYCLING

slightly to the next turn, a right at Via Coronel. Hit the rise here hard and you'll be rewarded with a quick roll through the next downhill. Be careful, though, there are three sizable speed bumps to prevent the Corvettes and Ferraris from achieving escape velocity. Coming out of a right-hand bend, you will see the road resume its climb at a consistent 8-percent grade; there's only a mile left to climb. You top out at Coronel Plaza, which is a large, square plot of grass, utterly devoid of trees . . . and shade. Finish off your water here because, once the descent begins, you won't have much opportunity to drink.

At Via Del Monte, turn left. The turns on this descent are uniformly easy, with one exception. Following a quick right–left bend combination, there is a tight right-hand switchback; brake fully for this before entering the turn. Take note of the signs saying stop ahead: there will be a stop sign immediately following your next right-hand bend; unprepared cyclists may encounter drivers entering the intersection. At the bottom of the runout, turn left onto Via Chico and pass back through the brick arch. Turn right onto Palos Verdes Drive West, and immediately move to the left lane to merge into Palos Verdes Boulevard. Once you are clear of the intersection, move back onto the shoulder.

Approximately 200 yards after the intersection, follow the left turn back onto Paseo de la Playa. Traffic approaching from the rear is likely to be traveling fast, so be extra careful as you cross the two lanes of traffic to the turn lane. After turning left onto Paseo de la Playa, take it directly back to Esplanade; you'll get one final ocean view before the end of the ride. At Esplanade, turn left and then immediately turn right onto Vista Del Mar, which delivers you back to the parking lot.

After the Ride
Exiting the parking lot, you are within walking distance of coffee shops and a variety of restaurants. From American fare to Mexican and French-style baked goods, you have many choices within 100 yards.

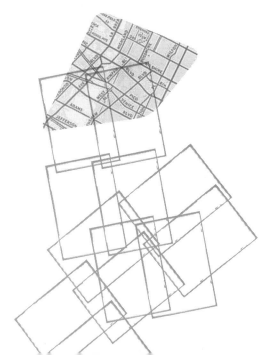

17 Lunada Bay Loop

AT A GLANCE

Length: 8 miles
Configuration: Loop
Difficulty: Easy
Climbing: 300 feet
Maximum gradient: 7%
Scenery: Ocean and the kind of homes that fill *Architectural Digest*
Exposure: Mornings are frequently overcast
Road traffic: Light
Road surface: Good
Riding time: 1 hour
Maps: Los Angeles County *Thomas Guide* pages 822 and 792

In Brief

This route combines some of the most lightly traveled roads in the South Bay and some of the prettiest coastline anywhere in the world. Views take in the cliffs of Lunada Bay, Catalina Island, and homes that are unaffordable to all but the biggest (and wealthiest) dreamers.

Directions

Located in Palos Verdes Estates, Lunada Bay is one of the more remote locations in Los Angeles County. From the I-10/I-405 interchange drive 12 miles south on I-405 and exit at Hawthorne Boulevard southbound. Drive south on Hawthorne 12.8 miles, until you reach Palos Verdes Drive South. At Palos Verdes, turn right, and drive 3 miles. At the intersection with Vista Del Mar (where the divided road ends), turn left into the parking lot overlooking the cliffs.

Description

As coastlines go, Palos Verdes has little trouble holding its own against some of the most notable coastlines touted in popular tourism guides. You name it: the Amalfi Coast, Big Sur, the Cinque Terre, this place is every bit as gorgeous . . . and it has one slight advantage. No one besides the locals have any reason to drive on the roads here. For reasons that can't be adequately explained, this is one area of LA that's completely devoid of looky-loo drivers.

Because the roads are so lightly traveled, this is one of the few rides in this guide that can be ridden nearly any time that's convenient to you, dear reader. There's a bit more traffic at rush hour, but most of these roads are residential, and Palos Verdes Drive South is the closest thing to a major thoroughfare on this route. This ride is very flat, and, although it's possible to do it on a beach cruiser, even a few gears will make the experience that much more enjoyable.

BICYCLING

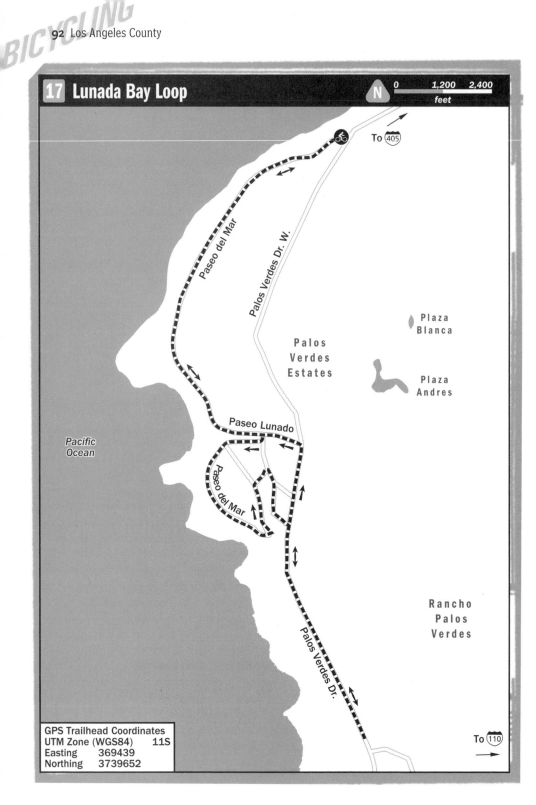

17 Lunada Bay Loop

N

0   1,200   2,400
feet

To 405

Paseo del Mar

Palos Verdes Dr. W.

Plaza Blanca

Plaza Andres

Palos Verdes Estates

Paseo Lunado

Pacific Ocean

Paseo del Mar

Rancho Palos Verdes

Palos Verdes Dr.

To 110

GPS Trailhead Coordinates
UTM Zone (WGS84)   11S
Easting   369439
Northing   3739652

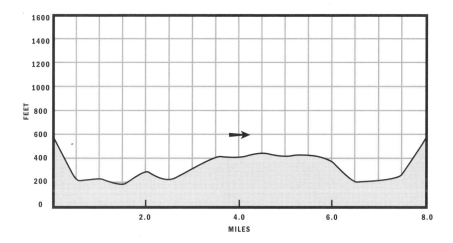

Families will be able to enjoy this ride with their teenagers quite easily.

The parking lot where you start has a commanding view of Bluff Cove, a well-known surf spot. Roll out of the parking lot and turn right onto Paseo Del Mar. Your first 1.5 miles are completely downhill and will give you a nice chance to spin your legs and begin warming up. Views of the coast will be somewhat intermittent here, gained only as land opens up between homes. Just past Via Bandini, the road turns up in its first hill on your route and becomes Paseo

Lunado. The hill is mercifully short (not quite a half-mile) and gentle in grade. What it does offer is a view of a small canyon that spills into Lunada Bay. The canyon splits Paseo Lunado in two, giving you extraordinary views of the homes on Resort Point across the way.

You will notice occasional signs identifying whale-watching observation points. In the winter, as the whales migrate, many pass within view of the Palos Verdes Peninsula because it juts into the Pacific. Whales can be sighted from the shore, thanks to the cliffs' elevation.

Turn right at Via Anacapa and immediately right again to head back down Paseo Lunado and past Resort Point. As you pass Lunada Bay School, you can be forgiven for wishing your parents hailed from Palos Verdes. The road changes back to Paseo Del Mar and begins to offer views of the coast again just past Via Neve. The road was reworked here a few years back after soil saturated by El Niño rains plunged into the ocean in terrific landslides. Some asphalt was lost along the way, but no homes took the plunge.

Resort Point juts into Lunada Bay and offers extraordinary views of the surrounding ocean.

The short kicker of a hill here is the steepest you encounter on this ride. It's not terribly steep, but if your bike is short on gears, it will require at least some effort. The road bends left and then intersects Via Alvarado. Turn left and take Via Alvarado one block to Via Sola. Climb Via Sola to Via Anacapa; climb Via Anacapa one block to Via Pacheco, and follow Via Pacheco one block as it bends to the right on its approach to Palos Verdes Drive South.

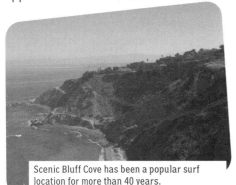
Scenic Bluff Cove has been a popular surf location for more than 40 years.

Turn right on Palos Verdes Drive South. There is a wide shoulder here that includes a bike lane. Some of the residents here feel less than charitable toward cyclists; as a result, the California Highway Patrol enforces the motor-vehicle codes affecting cyclists rather stringently. Stay to the right as much as possible. If you are alone or with a small group, you should have no problems staying right.

Almost immediately after turning right, you pass a home overlooking the bay with a large vineyard planted in the front yard. It's a great testament to the area's incredible climate that features warm days and cool nights.

Ride south on Palos Verdes Drive South 1.1 miles to Hawthorne Boulevard. Move into the left lane and, when you have a turn arrow, make a U-turn to head north again on Palos Verdes Drive. In the unlikely event you should want a short break, there is a shopping center on the southeast corner with a coffee shop.

This side of Palos Verdes Drive South also benefits from a wide shoulder and bike lane. The road is well swept, so staying to the right won't be a problem. Because your route here is slightly uphill, you'll have more opportunity to look across the road to the coast and take in views of Catalina Island. The rounded corner of the Palos Verdes Peninsula presents a constantly changing set of views; keep your eyes peeled.

At the 6-mile mark, after the stop sign halfway along Paseo Lunado, turn left onto the more northern half of that road. Here's your second big downhill of the day. Enjoy the easy spinning as you take in the coast. Paseo Del Mar guides you back to the parking lot where you started, but your ride will end with a bit of a challenge. Your longest climb of the day is the final mile of this ride, taking you back to the parking lot. The grade is gentle; relax and admire the homes around you.

After the Ride

In Rolling Hills Estates, atop the peninsula, there are a great many restaurants and shops, not to mention a mall with an ice-skating rink (in case the kids aren't tired yet). You might consider getting some takeout and driving back down Hawthorne Boulevard to Verde Ridge Road and having a picnic at Fred Hesse Community Park. High on the hill, the park offers views from Catalina to Orange County on clear days.

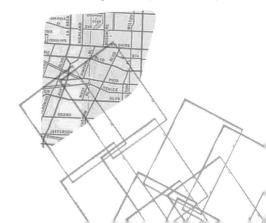

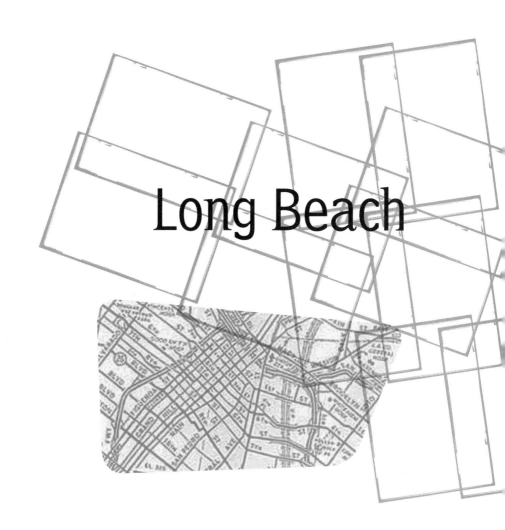

Long Beach

18 The Long Beach Bike Path

AT A GLANCE	**Length:** 6 miles (one way)
	Configuration: Out-and-back with spurs
	Difficulty: Easy
	Climbing: Less than 100 feet

Maximum gradient: 2%

Scenery: Beach, ocean, surfers galore, and the Long Beach skyline

Exposure: Mornings and late afternoons can be overcast

Road traffic: Very light

Road surface: Excellent

Riding time: 1 hour

Maps: Los Angeles County *Thomas Guide* page 825

In Brief

This ride is confined to the bike paths in the city of Long Beach and is wonderful for taking the whole family riding. There are a few street crossings that need to be managed and some riding alongside water in Rainbow Lagoon Park, but the riding is easy and family friendly. Also, if you are visiting from out of town and don't have a bike, you can rent one in Shoreline Village.

Directions

From the intersection of the I-405 and I-710, take I-710 southbound. When the 710 splits, giving you the choice of downtown or the Queen Mary, bear left toward downtown. Stay on the 710 until it ends at Shoreline Drive. Drive two blocks east on Shoreline and turn right onto Shoreline Village Drive. Turn right into the parking lot.

Description

From the parking lot at Shoreline Village, exit the parking lot to the west and ride up the ramp to the bike path. Immediately turn right and take the path north. The bike path in Long Beach takes a very circuitous route around the waterfront; it may seem a little disjointed, and you will double back on your path occasionally, but there are some beautiful vantages and serene sections of path. Almost immediately, the path turns right and crosses Shoreline Village Drive. Once across, turn left and take the path to the intersection with Shoreline Drive. Cross Shoreline Drive (there is a crossing button at the bike path) and turn left. This section of bike path follows the edge of a great deal of recent downtown development for Long Beach; riding here will feel like riding on sidewalks. The development is largely commercial, focusing on restaurants and shops.

The path turns left at Aquarium Way and crosses Shoreline Drive (again). The course parallels Aquarium Way and then turns

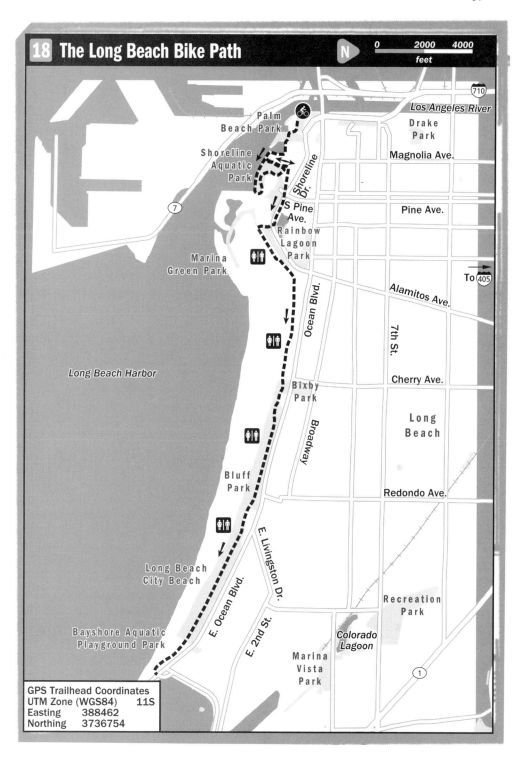

18 The Long Beach Bike Path

N

0   2000   4000
feet

Los Angeles River

710

Palm
Beach Park

Drake
Park

Magnolia Ave.

Shoreline
Aquatic
Park

Shoreline Dr.

Pine Ave.

7

S Pine
Ave.

Rainbow
Lagoon
Park

Marina
Green Park

Ocean Blvd.

Alamitos Ave.

To 405

Long Beach Harbor

7th St.

Cherry Ave.

Bixby
Park

Long
Beach

Broadway

Bluff
Park

Redondo Ave.

E. Livingston Dr.

Long Beach
City Beach

E. Ocean Blvd.

E. 2nd St.

Recreation
Park

Bayshore Aquatic
Playground Park

Colorado
Lagoon

Marina
Vista
Park

1

GPS Trailhead Coordinates
UTM Zone (WGS84)   11S
Easting   388462
Northing   3736754

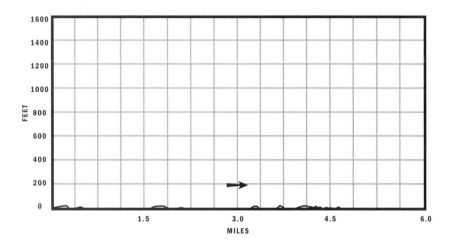

right under and passes beneath Queens Way. Your route now approaches Navy Landing, where the ferries depart to and arrive from Catalina Island. The path isn't well marked here. Follow the plaza to the left, and then watch for an opportunity to turn right. Immediately after turning right, the path markings will resume and indicate a left turn onto a stretch of path no wider than a sidewalk.

Pass Palm Beach Park. You will notice some wetlands here as you near the Los Angeles River. Ride up the short rise to the entrance to the Los Angeles Bikeway. From here, you may ride north up it. You can find a loop ride taking in the Bikeway on page 100.

Turn around and double back along Palm Beach Park and through Navy Landing. With the water now at your right, you may see one of the ferries departing or arriving at the dock. When you reach the underpass to Queens Way, continue straight on the bike path into Shoreline Park. Follow the curl of the path around the shore. At the next bike path intersection, make a sharp left

and spiral up the small rise to the observation tower. The view of Shoreline Village and downtown Long Beach from this slight elevation is worth soaking in.

Remount your bike and ride down the hill to rejoin the primary path. To your right is a small lagoon with several boat docks. The path will take you through a pedestrian plaza and by the Aquarium of the Pacific, a truly world-class institution. Be careful as you ride through this area. Although bicyclists are allowed to ride here, foot traffic is usually heavy on busy weekends, and avoiding all the pedestrians—who aren't likely to be watching for cyclists—can be a bit of a challenge.

As you approach the rotary at Aquarium Way, turn left and follow the bike path to the crossing. Next, cross Shoreline Drive and follow the path back toward the start, crossing Aquarium Way and South Pine Avenue. At Shoreline Village Drive, turn left and take in Rainbow Lagoon Park. The path hugs the lagoon and is a fun diversion. A word of caution: if you have small children, you might avoid this section. There are

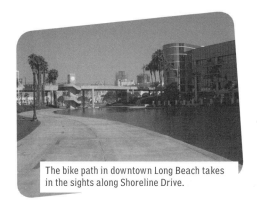

The bike path in downtown Long Beach takes in the sights along Shoreline Drive.

three bridges, which, while fun for adults, are a little too steep for children, and the lagoon itself has no guardrails. Come back when the little ones hit adolescence.

Back across East Shoreline Drive, follow the path south as it makes two left turns around the marina. The path takes you out to the end of the jetty, where you'll have a great view of Island Grisson, not to mention the hordes of sailboats waiting for the wind to kick up. Double back on the path, but when you reach Shoreline Village Drive this time continue straight on the path, hugging the edge of the marina.

Those who need restroom facilities may wonder why the first few buildings they see are restricted to sailors, but after leaving the marina you will see a succession of public restroom facilities on the bike path, affording plenty of opportunities for a pit stop.

At the end of the marina, the path makes a left then a right dogleg before proceeding out over the sand. Soon the path bends slightly left. You'll see the cliffhanging apartments to your left and the coast to your right. This stretch of coast is the domain of the kite surfers. Kite-surfing is where windsurfing and kite-flying meet. While that might sound redundant, to see it done well is to see something thrilling. However, for every kite surfer you see skittering over the surface of the water, you are likely to see three more standing on the beach just

trying to figure out how to play tug of war with a 747. They look for all the world like garden gnomes hanging from industrial-strength parasols in a tornado, which is to say that kite-surfing is fun to watch even when it's done poorly.

The path will end at the parking lot at Junipero Avenue. To join the next section of path, you must cross Junipero where it enters the beach parking lot. Watch for cars entering and exiting the lot; you'll see the path resume across the street.

At Belmont Pier, the path turns left and passes between some buildings on your left and a parking lot to your right. Cross South Termino Avenue and continue on the bike path through Olympic Plaza. Interestingly, the path passes to the *north* of the Belmont Plaza Pool through a grassy area lined with trees. At the east end of the aquatic center, turn right and follow the path back to the beach. From here it's just a mile to the end of the bike path. For those who aren't local, this part of Long Beach is called Belmont Shore, and it's a beautiful neighborhood worth exploring by bike. To get back to Shoreline Village, simply double back along the bike path and make sure to watch for the left–right dogleg past Belmont Plaza Pool.

After the Ride
You will probably have noticed the surreys along the path. These are two- or four-seat, four-wheeled, pedaled conveyances with a *Gilligan's Island* novelty to them. You might consider taking one out for a spin before you depart. There are plenty of restaurants in Shoreline Village and nearby at which you can refuel. As for other attractions in Long Beach, there are many. But if you have kids in tow (or if there's enough of a kid in you to be roused to wonder) make your way to the Aquarium of the Pacific.

The Los Angeles Bikeway Loop

AT A GLANCE

Length: 51 miles

Configuration: Loop

Difficulty: Moderate

Climbing: Less than 1,000 feet

Maximum gradient: 8%

Scenery: Beach, ocean, surfers galore, and the Long Beach skyline

Exposure: Mornings and late afternoons can be overcast

Road traffic: Moderate

Road surface: Excellent

Riding time: 3.5 hours

Maps: Los Angeles County *Thomas Guide*
pages 825, 795, 765, 735, 705, 706, 676, 636, 637, 677, 736, 766, 796, and 826

In Brief

There aren't a lot of places in central Los Angeles that offer riding that is both pretty and safe. This loop on three different bike paths offers a fascinating look at a more urban landscape. The bike path hugs three rivers: the Los Angeles, the Rio Hondo, and the San Gabriel. The ride passes through some communities that aren't considered the safest on the planet, but the bike paths themselves have maintained reputations as being safe for daytime recreation.

Directions

From the intersection of I-405 and I-710, take I-710 southbound. When the 710 splits, giving you the choice of downtown or the Queen Mary, bear left toward downtown. Stay on the 710 until it ends at Shoreline Drive. Drive two blocks east on Shoreline and turn right onto Shoreline Village Drive. Turn right into the parking lot.

Description

From the parking lot at Shoreline Village, exit west and ride up the ramp to the bike path. Immediately turn right and take the path north. The bike path in Long Beach takes a very circuitous route around the waterfront; these first few turns will seem a little odd. The path will turn right and cross Shoreline Village Drive. Immediately turn left and follow the path to the intersection with Shoreline Drive. Cross Shoreline Drive (there is a crossing button at the bike path) and turn left. This section of bike path follows the edge of a great deal of recent downtown Long Beach development; riding here will feel like riding on sidewalks. The development is largely commercial, focusing on restaurants and shops.

The path turns left at Aquarium Way and crosses Shoreline Drive (again). The course parallels Aquarium Way and then turns right under and passes beneath Queens Way. Your route now approaches Navy

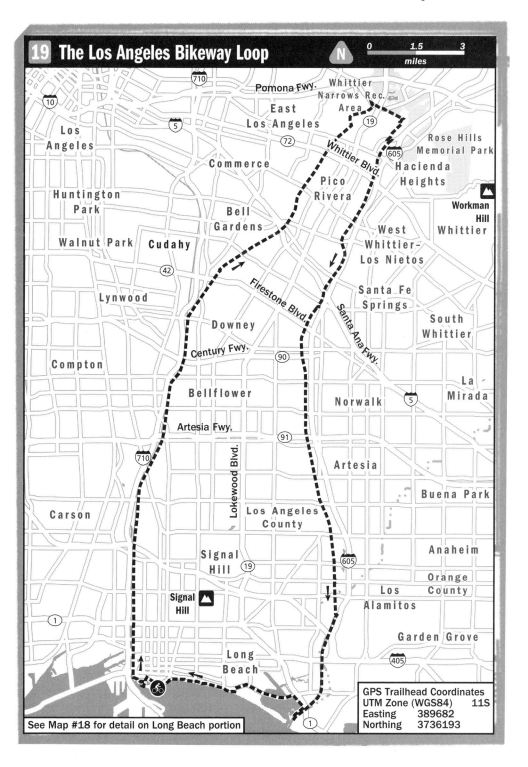

19 The Los Angeles Bikeway Loop

N

0   1.5   3
miles

710

Pomona Fwy.

Whittier Narrows Rec. Area

10

East Los Angeles

Los Angeles

5

19

72

605

Rose Hills Memorial Park

Commerce

Whittier Blvd.

Hacienda Heights

Pico Rivera

Huntington Park

Bell Gardens

Workman Hill Whittier

Walnut Park

Cudahy

West Whittier– Los Nietos

42

Lynwood

Firestone Blvd.

Santa Fe Springs

South Whittier

Downey

Santa Ana Fwy.

Compton

Century Fwy.

90

La Mirada

Bellflower

Norwalk

5

Artesia Fwy.

91

Artesia

710

Lokewood Blvd.

Buena Park

Carson

Los Angeles County

Signal Hill

19

605

Anaheim

Signal Hill

Orange County

Los Alamitos

1

Garden Grove

405

Long Beach

See Map #18 for detail on Long Beach portion

72

1

GPS Trailhead Coordinates
UTM Zone (WGS84)   11S
Easting   389682
Northing   3736193

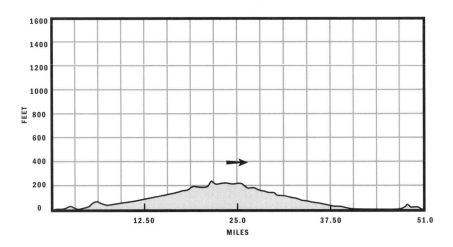

Landing, where the ferries depart to and arrive from Catalina Island. The path isn't well marked here. Follow the plaza to the left, and then watch for an opportunity to turn right. Immediately after turning right, the path markings will resume and indicate a left turn onto a stretch of path no wider than a sidewalk.

Pass Palm Beach Park. You will notice some wetlands here as you near the Los Angeles River. Ride up the short rise to the Los Angeles Bikeway and turn right. The Los Angeles River doesn't look like much of a river; in fact, it looks like a shipping channel. Further north, the river's banks are made from concrete and, well, it still doesn't look like a river. What it does look like is a location for a Hollywood action film, and you can be forgiven for making that association. A great many action classics filmed pivotal sequences here, including *Terminator 2* and the remake of *The Italian Job*.

The section of the Los Angeles Bikeway you are riding on is 12 miles long. The scenery to your left is riverine. And to your right is a constantly evolving landscape of industrial and suburban development with a few unusual sights thrown in, including a golf course in Compton. Just before the Rio Hondo River feeds into the Los Angeles River, there is a bridge. Here the Los Angeles Bikeway turns left and continues north along the river as the Rio Hondo Bike Path. Shortly after the Los Angeles River splits from the Rio Hondo River (you are riding upstream), you will encounter a bridge crossing the Rio Hondo. Turn left to cross the bridge, and immediately turn right to continue northeast along the Rio Hondo Bike Path.

The Rio Hondo Bike Path passes through a largely Latino part of Los Angeles. The views here are full of surprises. Although the river bed may be concrete and the water flow for much of the year is token, there are still many great sights. No one is likely to get excited about all the crows and pigeons, but if you keep your eyes peeled you can see mallard ducks, Canada geese (in winter), white egrets, and red-tailed hawks. Rabbits will occasionally dart across the path. This area is also a popular with equestrians.

There are trails that line the path, and you will see residents riding horses.

Arguably the greatest hazard you will encounter during your ride will be broken glass on the path. Broken beer bottles aren't common, but you are likely to find one or two on your ride. The major-artery underpasses seem to be among the most popular spots for nighttime drinking.

The Rio Hondo Bike Path passes under eight larger streets in the space of 7 miles before arriving at the Whittier Narrows Dam. The path will turn sharply left, and you'll encounter one of the steepest hills of the entire ride; fortunately, it is only about 50 yards long. The path will continue to the north before passing through some fencing (to prevent unauthorized cars from driving onto the dam). Turn right and pass between a gate and guardrail to resume your course. The path drops down the other side of the dam into the flood-control basin. The basin has been left wild, and the combination of trees and shrubs is a refreshing switch. The path ends at Lincoln Avenue. Turn right on Lincoln and immediately right again onto San Gabriel Boulevard. This will be one of only two stretches of road on this ride.

In winter and spring when the rain comes, this area may become flooded. If that's the case, instead of riding down-hill into the basin, continue to Lincoln Avenue and turn right. Lincoln will take you to San Gabriel Boulevard, where you rejoin your course.

San Gabriel Boulevard crosses Rose-mead Boulevard and becomes Durfee Avenue. At Siphon Road, exit Durfee and ride up the ramp to join the San Gabriel River Bike Path. Siphon Road will seem like a bike path more than a road (mainly because it looks like one and there won't be any cars on it). Ride east 0.75 miles and turn left onto the San Gabriel River Bike Trail. Only 100 meters from the turn, you will ride back up the Whittier Narrows Dam. There is a sharp left turn at the bottom of the hill; be careful not to take the turn too quickly because there is often some sand on the path here. At the top of the dam, the path cuts to the right briefly before continuing down the other side.

Just more than a half-mile from the dam, the path does something a little odd: A ramp will send you up to San Gabriel River Parkway. To continue south on the bike path, you must turn left and ride oppo-site the flow of traffic on the shoulder. As strange as this may seem, this is the only way to continue on the ride; fortunately, the shoulder is wide. The purpose here is to get to the other side of the river, and this is the easiest way for cyclists to get across the bridge. Once you have crossed the bridge, turn left. You may wish to walk—rather than ride—down a rather steep ramp to pass beneath San Gabriel River Parkway.

Except at the San Gabriel River Parkway, the San Gabriel River Bike Trail will pass under major thoroughfares the same way the Rio Hondo Bike Path does, but there are two places where the underpass is rather narrow and dark. As you enter underpasses, announce your presence.

Seven miles after turning onto the San Gabriel River Bike Trail, you will encounter a public park on your left. Wilderness Park (not exactly an accurate name) affords a

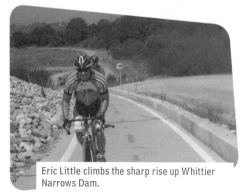

Eric Little climbs the sharp rise up Whittier Narrows Dam.

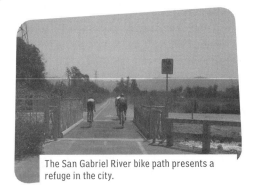

The San Gabriel River bike path presents a refuge in the city.

great opportunity to top off your water bottles and use the restroom if you have to answer the call of nature. Should you wish to pass up this opportunity, you will encounter Liberty Park 5.8 miles along. Another 2.6 miles south on the San Gabriel River Bike Trail, you will enter El Dorado Park. This is a very large park and well worth devoting a visit.

As you continue south, you will notice that the riverside development changes, seeming to go from residential one minute to industrial the next. Much of the change reflects differences in zoning regulations from community to community.

The bike path comes to an end at Regatta Way. It may come as little surprise that you have returned to the coast and are entering a marina. For the next 3.2 miles, you must ride on city streets. Technically, you are just inside Orange County at this point, but only by 100 yards or so. Turn right on Regatta Way, cross the bridge over the San Gabriel River, and then immediately turn right on North Marina Drive, which will travel north for a little more than 100 yards before bending left and becoming East Marina Drive.

Turn left at East Second Street and cross the bridge to Naples Island. Naples is a tiny island (0.7 miles across) with a number of restaurants and shops and a fair selection of trophy homes. You will leave Naples Island via another bridge, cross Alamitos Bay, and

enter the Long Beach neighborhood known as Belmont Shore.

Turn left on East Livingston Drive and ride 0.4 miles to Termino Avenue. Move into the left lane and turn. Termino Avenue will intersect East Allin Street. Ride one block to the Belmont Pier, then turn left and ride up the ramp. You will see markings directing you to the bike path to your right. This final section of bike path is 2.6 miles long.

Among the more amusing sights here are of people riding surreys, which can be rented near Shoreline Village. A surrey is a four-person, pedaled conveyance with a tasseled top and a *Flintstones* sense of style. If you are there in the afternoon, you'll see people kite surfing; it is quite a marvel to watch.

After the Ride

Shoreline Village is a little touristy but has some good restaurants, not to mention some casual options for coffee and pastries. If you'd like more choices, cross Shoreline Drive to the development along The Promenade.

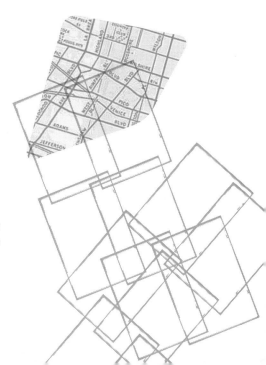

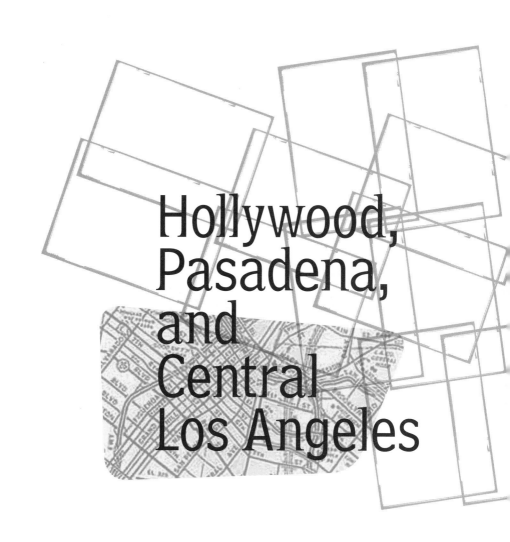

Hollywood, Pasadena, and Central Los Angeles

20 El Dorado Park

AT A GLANCE

Length: 4 miles
Configuration: Loop
Difficulty: Easy
Climbing: Less than 25 feet

Maximum gradient: 2%

Scenery: Palm trees, grassy fields, and wetlands

Exposure: Plenty of shade from trees on the bike path

Road traffic: Light

Road surface: Good to excellent

Riding time: 30 minutes

Maps: Los Angeles County *Thomas Guide* pages 766 and 796

In Brief

El Dorado Park is one of the hidden gems of Los Angeles (Long Beach, in fact) that help make it a more livable place than many people imagine. The route here covers a few roads and some bike paths that keep riders away from the crush of the city. This short ride can be enjoyed with family, but it's also a great training spot for the ambitious cyclist. Entrance to the park costs $4. If you want, bring a picnic lunch and plan to enjoy the area's other attractions after your ride.

Directions

From the South Bay: From the intersection of I-405 and I-105, drive 20.5 miles south on the 405. Exit at Studebaker Road, turn left, and drive 1.4 miles to East Spring Street. Turn right and go 0.8 miles to the entrance to El Dorado Park on your left.

From downtown: From the intersection of I-5 and US 101, drive 9.75 miles south on I-5 to I-605. Merge onto the 605 and continue south another 9.4 miles. Exit at Spring Street, bear right at the bottom of the ramp, and immediately turn right into El Dorado Park.

Description

There aren't many rides in this guide that aren't time dependent. That is, most of them are safer and more enjoyable if you ride earlier in the day. This ride is a notable exception. Because the entire course is located within a 400-square-acre Long Beach city park, traffic is always minimal.

El Dorado Park is pancake flat, provided you don't mind a pancake with a few ripples, which is to say its not being completely level is more accidental than intentional. The park is at the eastern edge of Long Beach, where Los Angeles County abuts Orange County. The geography here is remarkably flat, compared with other areas of LA County (and many locations featured in this guide).

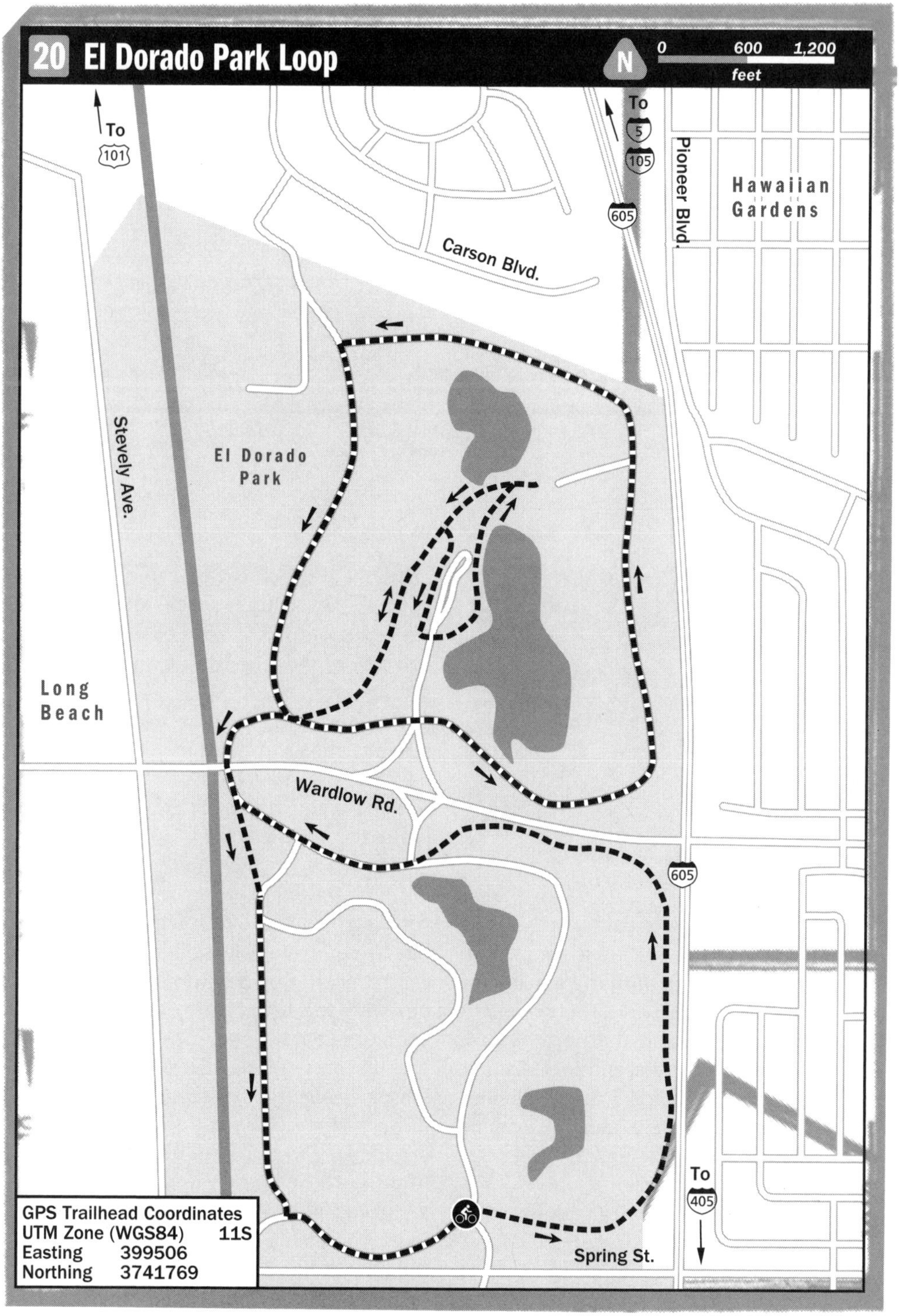

20 **El Dorado Park Loop**

N

0   600   1,200
feet

To
101

To
5
105

605

Pioneer Blvd.

Carson Blvd.

Hawaiian
Gardens

Stevely Ave.

El Dorado
Park

Long
Beach

Wardlow Rd.

605

Spring St.

To
405

GPS Trailhead Coordinates
UTM Zone (WGS84)   11S
Easting   399506
Northing   3741769

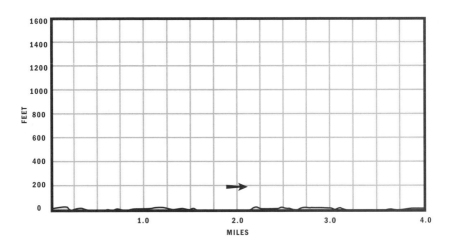

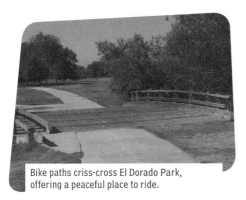

Bike paths criss-cross El Dorado Park, offering a peaceful place to ride.

This ride is actually composed of two different loops. The first is a simple 1.9-mile ride on a bike path that encircles the southern half of the park. The second is a 1.7-mile road loop at the north end of the park, away from the entrance. This is the site of the El Dorado Park race series, which takes place every Tuesday evening from March through August. There are several categories of racing; more information about the series can be found at **www.californiabicycleracing.org**.

For families looking for a safe place to ride with children, away from throngs of people and the threat of traffic, El Dorado Park is ideal. Its suburban location is convenient to much of Los Angeles, but because of the single entrance there is no through traffic.

After entering the park, either continue straight ahead to the northern end of the park for the road loop or, if you wish to ride the bike path, just park at the side of the road.

There are entrances to the bike path just north of the main entrance to the park. If you begin to the right of the entrance to ride a counterclockwise loop, your route will parallel I-605 briefly. It's a little noisy, but with the lush, grassy meadow, you'll soon tune out the sound.

The path gradually bears left along Wardlow Avenue, which divides the park in half. There is a road crossing, but you are unlikely to encounter any traffic here. Another 50 meters on, you will encounter a second road crossing. At this point, the path crosses the road that passes beneath the tunnel under Wardlow Avenue. To continue on the path, cross the street and turn left. If you turn right, that will take you into the northern part of the park. There is an alternative, which is to bear left on the path and exit onto the San Gabriel River Bike Path. That path actually passes through the park briefly; should you wish to go on a longer ride, the San Gabriel River Bike Path extends for miles both north and south of the park. Additionally, there are sections of bike path within the northern half of the park. They do not form any sort of continuous loop, however.

Continue on the path that parallels the river bike path. The concrete ribbon threads through trees that bathe riders in shade. The lazy arc returns to the park entrance following a final bend just before the gate.

Riders interested in a little more strenuous workout without the hassle of traffic should head to one of the parking areas at the north end of the park, beyond the tunnel under Wardlow Avenue. The race series has an official start/finish roughly 0.8 miles from the first parking area beyond the tunnel. Riders generally ride the course in a counterclockwise loop, just as the race series does.

Though the loop is bowling-alley flat, experienced riders will note the challenge the wind poses. For much of the day, an offshore breeze pushes through the park from the west. On the straight, eastern stretch of the loop, the crosswind isn't too noticeable. But as the road curls left around one of the park's ponds, the wind gradually becomes a headwind and presents a real challenge.

The first turn of the loop is a long sweeper. Stay on the gas here; you'll never scrape a pedal. The second turn is significantly sharper. Set up far to the right and apex late to pedal through the turn; try as they might, many riders cannot pedal through this turn. As the road cuts back to the left, there is a small dip followed by a rise into the headwind. Gut your way

through the dip and then gradually bend into the right that follows. As you near the parking lot, the road curves to the left once again and then sweeps into the third turn. Upon exiting that turn, stand up and shift up a cog; the wind at your back gives you just the nudge you need to generate some more speed. The road twists through a lazy right–left chicane before entering the fourth turn for the drag race to the start/finish line.

After the Ride

Before loading up the car and heading out, take a stroll around any one of the park's many ponds. This is a surprisingly serene location, given its position in the city. For kids (of all ages), there are train rides, pony rides, hayrides, and a petting zoo. Other park attractions include an archery range, model plane and sailboat areas, a nature center, a 12-station physical-fitness course, picnic areas (some with shelters), and playgrounds.

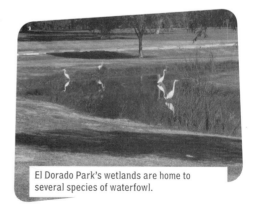

El Dorado Park's wetlands are home to several species of waterfowl.

21 Griffith Park Loop

AT A GLANCE

Length: 8 miles

Configuration: Loop

Difficulty: Moderate

Climbing: 400 feet

Maximum gradient: 7%

Scenery: Golf course, picnic areas, tree-lined roads

Exposure: There is some occasional shade afforded by the trees

Road traffic: Light

Road surface: Good

Riding time: 45 minutes

Maps: Los Angeles County *Thomas Guide* pages 594, 564, and 563

In Brief

This loop through Griffith Park is a gentle and easy ride through one of LA's premiere leisure spots. The ride takes you by a golf course, several picnic areas, the Los Angeles Zoo, the Autry National Center, and Travel Town, a museum devoted to train travel.

Directions

From the interchange of I-5 and I-110, travel north on I-5 and exit at Crystal Springs Road/Griffith Park. From the ramp, turn left on Crystal Springs. A quarter-mile south on Crystal Springs, make a U-turn after the median; there will be a sign directing you to the Griffith Park train and the pony rides. Just after the U-turn, you will see the parking lot on the right.

Description

From the parking lot, exit to the north on Crystal Springs Road. For much of the loop, there is a painted shoulder at the right of the road. Initially, the road parallels I-5 before veering away and around the golf course. The two-lane road features wide lanes with gentle bends.

The road will climb very, very gently, usually about 0.5 to 1 percent. At 2 miles, the road will bend to the right, and a parking lot will spread alongside you on your left. The road becomes Western Heritage Way. Following a curve to the left, you pass between the Los Angeles Zoo (on your left) and the Autry National Center (on your right); the latter takes its name from the Western star Gene Autry.

Just beyond the intersection at Zoo Drive (where most visitors to the zoo and the Autry Center exit the 5), the road bends left to parallel CA 134 (the Hollywood Freeway). Fortunately, the park is shielded to some degree from the freeway by a stand of trees that blocks a direct view of it and helps cut down on noise pollution as well. This is the northern edge of the park; hills rise to

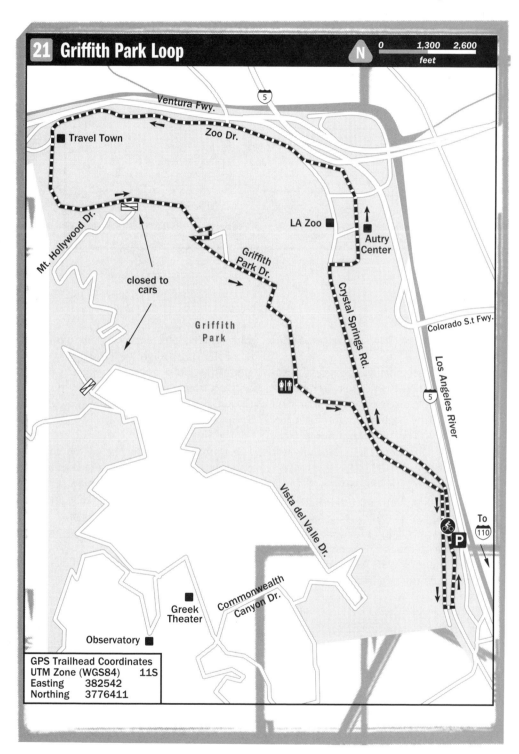

21 Griffith Park Loop

N

0   1,300   2,600
feet

Ventura Fwy.

5

Zoo Dr.

■ Travel Town

Mt. Hollywood Dr.

closed to cars

Griffith Park Dr.

LA Zoo ■

■
Autry
Center

Crystal Springs Rd.

Colorado S.t Fwy.

Griffith
Park

Los Angeles River

5

Vista del Valle Dr.

To
110

P

Greek
Theater ■

Commonwealth
Canyon Dr.

Observatory ■

GPS Trailhead Coordinates
UTM Zone (WGS84)   11S
Easting   382542
Northing   3776411

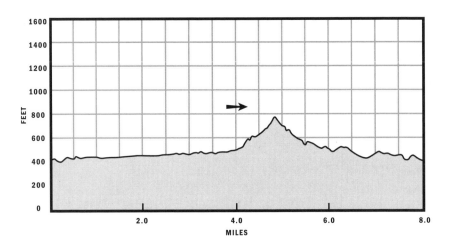

the left. Western Heritage Way becomes Zoo Drive here.

At 4 miles—the halfway point in the ride —you reach Travel Town, a railway museum known for its old engines and Pullman cars. Zoo Drive curls around Travel Town and meets Griffith Park Drive. Continue straight, onto Griffith Park Drive; do not turn right to continue on Zoo Drive.

After crossing the intersection, the road begins climbing the only real hill of the entire ride. It rises nearly 300 feet in 1.7 miles for an average gradient of 3 percent. It's a gentle climb that takes you, finally, into the interior of the park. Horse trails line the road and lead into the woods that surround it.

On the descent, you pass two different picnic areas, one of which has a playground and bathrooms. The descent is technically easy, with one exception. Just over a half-mile into the descent, there is a tight right turn; brake early and you'll be fine.

As the downhill flattens out, you pass the clubhouse for the golf course. Watch traffic pulling into the road from the two

parking lots, one each on your right and left. Following a slight rise, there is another gentle descent of approximately 0.25 miles. At the runout, Griffith Park Drive intersects Crystal Springs. Turn right onto Crystal Springs.

The final 1.3 miles of the ride roll over two slight hills. At the top of the second one, you will see the sign for the U-turn that will take you around the median dividing the road and back to the parking area for the pony rides and train ride.

After the Ride
If you have children, the train and the pony rides can be a lot of fun. There is a snack bar, and during the summer there is a concession for sno-cones and popsicles. The Autry Center, the LA Zoo, and Travel Town are fun whether or not you have children.

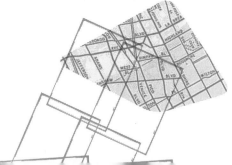

22 Griffith Park Observatory Loop

AT A GLANCE

Length: 20 miles

Configuration: Loop

Difficulty: Moderate

Climbing: 2,200 feet

Maximum gradient: 8%

Scenery: Golf course, picnic areas, views of the San Fernando Valley, wooded areas, Griffith Park Observatory, the Hollywood sign, views of downtown

Exposure: Mornings and late afternoons can be overcast

Road traffic: Moderate

Road surface: OK

Riding time: 2 hours

Maps: Los Angeles County *Thomas Guide* pages 594, 564, 563, and 593

In Brief

This longer loop through Griffith Park will take you by the features found in the shorter loop, including the LA Zoo, the Autry National Center, Travel Town, and the golf course and picnic areas. The ride's most distinguishing feature, however, is the network of roads that are inaccessible by cars. They offer rare and beautiful views of the city. The recently refurbished Griffith Park Observatory crowns the ride.

Directions

From the interchange of I-5 and I-110, travel north on I-5 and exit at Crystal Springs Road/Griffith Park. From the ramp, turn left on Crystal Springs. A quarter-mile south on Crystal Springs, make a U-turn after the median; there will be a sign directing you to the Griffith Park train and the pony rides. Just after the U-turn, you will see the parking lot on the right.

Description

From the parking lot, exit to the north on Crystal Springs Road. For much of the loop, there is a painted shoulder at the right of the road. Initially, the road parallels I-5 before veering away and around the golf course. The two-lane road features wide lanes with gentle bends.

The road will climb very, very gently,

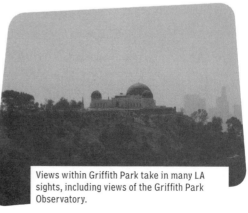

Views within Griffith Park take in many LA sights, including views of the Griffith Park Observatory.

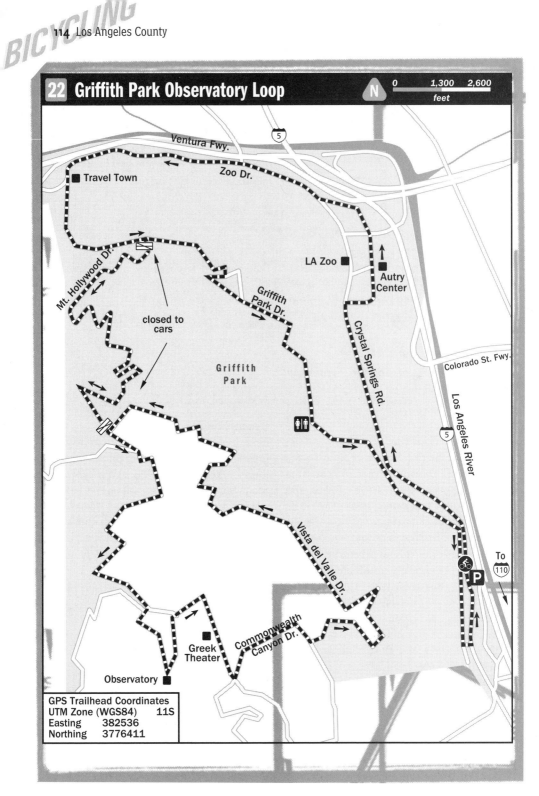

BICYCLING

N

0   1,300   2,600
feet

Ventura Fwy.

5

Zoo Dr.

Travel Town

Mt. Hollywood Dr.

closed to cars

Griffith Park Dr.

LA Zoo

Autry Center

Crystal Springs Rd.

Colorado St. Fwy.

Griffith Park

Los Angeles River

5

Vista del Valle Dr.

To
110

Commonwealth Canyon Dr.

Greek Theater

Observatory

GPS Trailhead Coordinates
UTM Zone (WGS84)   11S
Easting   382536
Northing   3776411

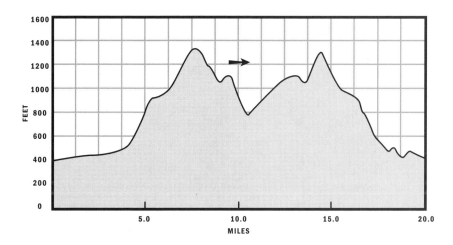

usually about 0.5 to 1 percent. At 2 miles, the road will bend to the right, and a parking lot will spread alongside you on your left. The road becomes Western Heritage Way. Following a curve to the left, you pass between the Los Angeles Zoo (on your left) and the Autry National Center (on your right); the latter takes its name from the Western star Gene Autry.

Just beyond the intersection at Zoo Drive (where most visitors to the zoo and the Autry Center exit I-5), the road bends left to parallel CA 134 (the Hollywood Freeway). Fortunately, the park is shielded to some degree from the freeway by a stand of trees that blocks a direct view of it and helps cut down on noise pollution as well. This is the northern edge of the park; hills rise to the left. Western Heritage Way becomes Zoo Drive here.

At 4 miles—the halfway point in the ride—you reach Travel Town, a railway museum known for its old engines and Pullman cars. Zoo Drive curls around Travel Town and meets Griffith Park Drive. Continue straight, onto Griffith Park Drive; do not turn right to continue on Zoo Drive.

After crossing the intersection, the road begins climbing, rising nearly 300 feet in 1.7 miles for an average gradient of 3 percent. Just before the top, there is an intersection and a gate at the right. The two arms of the gate are chained and locked to prevent cars from making the right turn onto Mount Hollywood Drive. Dismount your bike and step over the gate to resume your ride.

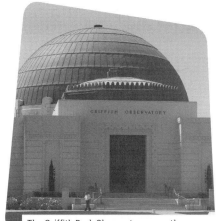

The Griffith Park Observatory recently received a multi-million dollar restoration.

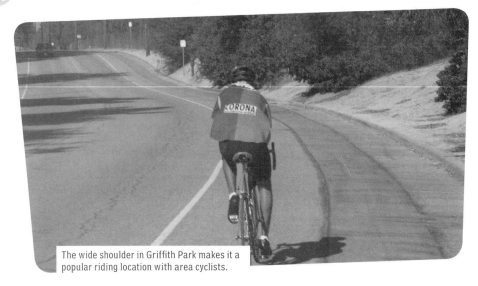

The wide shoulder in Griffith Park makes it a popular riding location with area cyclists.

Mount Hollywood will take you deep into the interior of the park. Most of the roads here haven't received much maintenance in recent history. The surface is OK for the most part, but there are sections covered by a layer of dirt and/or sand. Any time you can't see the road surface, exercise caution. At the time of this writing, there was one short section where a hillside was being reinforced and the road surface was gravel; it comes within a half-mile of resuming the climb following the gate.

Initially, the views on the climb are to the north, looking into Burbank and Glendale. Generally, the grade is rather slight—almost never more than 4 percent. The road twists, bends, and curls unendingly; new vistas are constant, making the climb one of the most unceasingly interesting in this guide. Roughly 6.4 miles in, you round a bend and, across the canyon at your right, you will see a sidelong view of the Hollywood sign. As you continue around the next few bends, the view improves.

At the top of the climb, Mount Hollywood intersects Vista Del Valle Drive. Stay to the right and begin to descend. Next, Mount Hollywood will intersect Griffith Park.

Continue your descent straight on Mount Hollywood. A gate seals Mount Hollywood Drive from traffic at this end. Brake carefully as you descend the final yards to the gate. Mount Hollywood ends here at the intersection of Vermont Canyon Road and East Observatory Avenue. Turn right on East Observatory and begin the brief climb up to Griffith Park Observatory.

Don't be surprised if the observatory grounds look familiar to you even if you've never been here before. The site has been used in many movies, including *The Terminator*, *The Rocketeer*, and, most significantly, the final scenes of *Rebel Without a Cause*. A bust of James Dean stands on the front lawn.

Descend from the observatory to Vermont Canyon Road. Turn right on Vermont Canyon and continue to descend. Following a right switchback, you will come upon the Greek Theater, which is arguably one of the best places to see live music in all of Los Angeles. The site is beautiful, and the acoustics unusually good. As you pass the theater, begin watching for an opportunity to turn left. Commonwealth Canyon Drive is easy to miss amid the theater parking areas.

Commonwealth Canyon immediately kicks up a steep hill; while it's not long, it's a bit too steep for most to push over in the big ring. Fortunately, the road flattens out until your next turn. At Vista Del Valle Drive, turn left for the climb back up to Mount Hollywood. The ascent is roughly 3.5 miles long, and the final mile includes the steepest section of over a half-mile, averaging 8.5 percent.

Vista Del Valle intersects Mount Hollywood. The junction should look familiar. Turn right and begin your descent back to the gate at Griffith Park Drive, but be mindful of the section of gravel at the retaining wall. It comes up following two brief bends, the first to the right and the next to the left; you will be able to see the retaining wall before you reach it. Less than a half mile later, after rounding a right bend, stop, dismount, and step over the gate. After remounting your bike, continue over the slight rise to the top of Griffith Park Drive and descend by the picnic areas, one of which has a playground and bathrooms.

As the downhill flattens out, you pass the clubhouse for the golf course. Watch traffic pulling into the road from the two parking lots—one each on your right and left. Following a slight rise, there is another gentle descent of approximately 0.25 miles. At the runout, Griffith Park Drive intersects Crystal Springs. Turn right onto Crystal Springs Road.

The final 1.3 miles of the ride roll over two slight hills. At the top of the second one, you will see the sign for the U-turn that will take you around the median dividing the road and back to the parking area for the pony rides and train ride.

After the Ride

If you have children, the train and the pony rides can be a lot of fun. There is a snack bar, and during the summer there is a concession for sno-cones and popsicles. The Autry Center, the LA Zoo, and Travel Town are fun whether or not you have children. Griffith Park Observatory shows are a great way to spend leisure time, and the Greek Theater can make for an excellent evening.

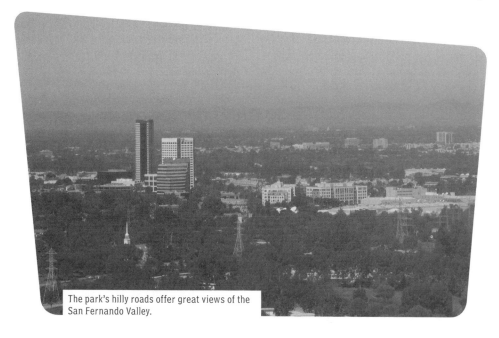

The park's hilly roads offer great views of the San Fernando Valley.

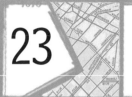

23 Hollywood Landmarks

AT A GLANCE	**Length:** 9 miles
	Configuration: Loop
	Difficulty: Easy
	Climbing: 300 feet

Maximum gradient: 5%

Scenery: Famous movie landmarks

Exposure: No shade, except for the odd building shadow

Road traffic: Heavy, except on weekend mornings

Road surface: Fair

Riding time: 1 hour

Maps: Los Angeles County *Thomas Guide* pages 592 and 593

In Brief

This tour of Hollywood and the Sunset Strip gives you the opportunity to get a sense of Hollywood as a community, where the famous cinemas, hotels, and restaurants are all woven into the fabric of daily existence. It's hard to get this sense from a car, and on foot it is impossible. Even for those who have never heard the siren call of Hollywood, after riding these streets you can understand the mythical pull this place has on performers, writers, and directors.

Directions

From I-405, exit Sunset Boulevard East and drive 5.75 miles to West Hollywood. After passing Doheny Drive, turn on any of the side streets to look for free street parking. Alternatively, there is metered parking on Sunset Boulevard. From US 101, exit Sunset Boulevard West and drive 4.5 miles to Larrabee Street, then begin looking for parking.

Description

The majority of this ride is built around a 4-mile stretch of Sunset Boulevard. Along with New York's Park Avenue and Paris's Champs-Elysées, Sunset is arguably one of the most famous streets in the world. As the epicenter of the American entertainment industry, it is at once both the fantasy "easy street" and the reality of the "boulevard of broken dreams."

This ride offers little in the way of challenges for the rider, and road conditions are nothing to write home about. However, even for residents of Southern California, this ride offers a panorama that any movie watcher will recognize. Even the most jaded antiestablishment, tabloidphobic, art-house aesthete will be impressed with this ride's glimpses of places for which you can't help but experience some fondness and nostalgia.

As with many rides in this guide, there is a limited window during which you may

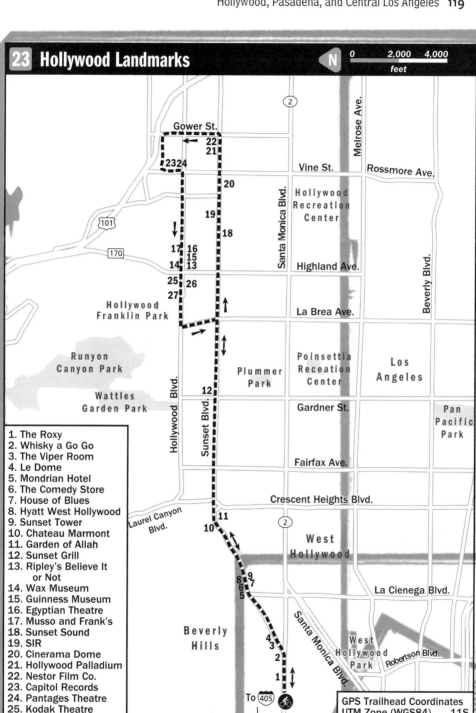

23 Hollywood Landmarks

N

0   2,000   4,000
feet

Gower St.

22
21

2324

20

Vine St.

Rossmore Ave.

Melrose Ave.

19

18

Santa Monica Blvd.

Hollywood
Recreation
Center

17 16
    15
14 13

Highland Ave.

Beverly Blvd.

25 26
27

Hollywood
Franklin Park

La Brea Ave.

Runyon
Canyon Park

Plummer
Park

Poinsettia
Receation
Center

Los
Angeles

Wattles
Garden Park

Hollywood Blvd.

Sunset Blvd.

12

Gardner St.

Pan
Pacific
Park

1. The Roxy
2. Whisky a Go Go
3. The Viper Room
4. Le Dome
5. Mondrian Hotel
6. The Comedy Store
7. House of Blues
8. Hyatt West Hollywood
9. Sunset Tower
10. Chateau Marmont
11. Garden of Allah
12. Sunset Grill
13. Ripley's Believe It
    or Not
14. Wax Museum
15. Guinness Museum
16. Egyptian Theatre
17. Musso and Frank's
18. Sunset Sound
19. SIR
20. Cinerama Dome
21. Hollywood Palladium
22. Nestor Film Co.
23. Capitol Records
24. Pantages Theatre
25. Kodak Theatre
26. El Capitan Theatre
27. Grauman's Chinese

Fairfax Ave.

Crescent Heights Blvd.

11

Laurel Canyon
Blvd.

10

West
Hollywood

8 9
6 7
5

La Cienega Blvd.

Beverly
Hills

4
3
2

1

Santa Monica Blvd.

West
Hollywood
Park

Robertson Blvd.

To 405

GPS Trailhead Coordinates
UTM Zone (WGS84)   11S
Easting   371822
Northing   3773049

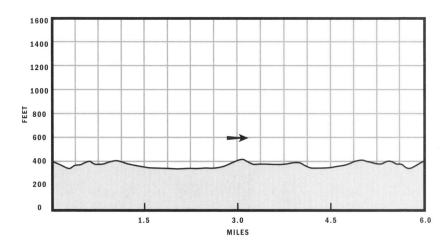

enjoy the journey; Saturday and Sunday mornings are your only shot. While everyone is sleeping off the previous night's revelry, you get a brief opportunity to cruise the streets without concern for the drunken starlets in their six-figure SUVs. Carpe diem, dude.

From the corner of Sunset and Doheny Drive, begin riding east on Sunset. You needn't pedal far to reach your first landmark: The Roxy. Located at 9009 Sunset (on the north side), it is known as one of *the* locations for emerging talent, it's not uncommon to see a star in the crowd checking out the latest sounds. Just two blocks on is the Whisky a Go Go (8901). Played by the likes of The Doors, Janice Joplin, and Led Zeppelin, it is also known as the birthplace of go-go dancing. A block further, on the south side, at 8852, is Johnny Depp's club, The Viper Room.

Sunset bends left and begins to climb slightly. On the left is Le Dome (8720), a very popular spot for an industry power lunch. Half a mile further is a concentrated stretch of Sunset glory. The Mondrian

Hotel (8440) has hosted everyone from The Who to Smashing Pumpkins, and the hotel's Sky Bar is said to be a who's who of current celebritydom. Next door (8430) is the House of Blues, which, while lacking the history of a place like The Whisky, regularly hosts some very big acts giving

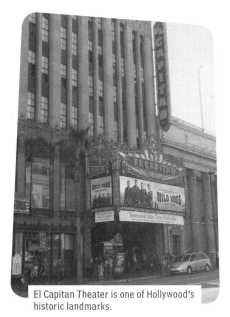

El Capitan Theater is one of Hollywood's historic landmarks.

intimate performances. Across the street (8433), The Comedy Store is the place all comics hope to go when they die. You haven't made it until you've played this place. Back across the street (8401) is the Hyatt West Hollywood. Once affectionately nicknamed the "Riot House," it served as a home away from home for many of the top stars of the 1970s, especially Led Zeppelin. In Little Richard's case, it simply served as home for most of the 1980s and 1990s. Back across the street, at 8358, is the former Sunset Tower Hotel, now called The Argyle. This gem of Art Deco architecture was once home to Clark Gable, John Wayne, and Marilyn Monroe, among others. More recently, it has appeared in *Get Shorty*, *Guilty by Suspicion*, and the Hollywood satire *The Player*.

Almost a half-mile farther, just past Harper Avenue, on the north side of Sunset at 8221, is Chateau Marmont. This is the place that stars who don't have an LA home stay when they are here for extended periods. Its guest list is a laundry list of famous names. One block farther on the south side is the former site of the Garden of Allah (8152), the place Joni Mitchell memorialized in the song "Big Yellow Taxi" with the line: "They paved paradise and put up a parking lot."

At 2.25 miles you cross Gardner Street, and on the north side at 7439 is the Sunset Grill, a spot popular enough with stars to be immortalized in a Don Henley song. Across the street is one of the most famous recording studios in the world: the Sound Factory; while its big brother around the corner on Selma—Sunset Sound—might boast some bigger names, Sound Factory has a client list that Lollapalooza would envy: Toto, Crowded House, Carole King, Little Feat, Warren Zevon, Elvis Costello, and Sheryl Crow, just for starters. Chances are, no matter what kind of music you

This tour of Hollywood and the Sunset Strip gives you the opportunity to get a sense of Hollywood as a community, where the famous cinemas, hotels, and restaurants are all woven into the fabric of daily existence.

listen to, some artist in your collection recorded here.

Another three blocks on at 6465 is Studio Instrument Rental. Aside from giving you the opportunity to play a real gold-top Les Paul or a Hammond B-3, this place has served as the rehearsal space for many acts.

In the 1960s, filmmaking took an unconventional turn when Cinerama was introduced; involving projection onto three screens, it was Imax before there was Imax. The original Cinerama Dome is at 6360 and continues to show movies today. Three blocks up (6215) is the Hollywood Palladium, once the world's largest dance club. Another block on (6121) is KCBS-TV, once the site of Nestor Film Company, the very first film studio to set up shop in Hollywood.

Turn left at Gower Street and begin pedaling uphill. This is the biggest hill of the ride. A little more than 0.3 miles later, turn left at Yucca Street, which comes just before the 101. Three blocks on, turn left on Vine Street. On your left is the Capitol Records building. At the intersection of Hollywood Boulevard, look to your left before turning. East of the intersection is the Art Deco Pantages Theatre, still used for a great many movie premieres and theatrical productions.

Turn right and begin pedaling west on Hollywood Boulevard. To your right is the Hollywood Walk of Fame. Not all the stars here have transcended time. Sure, everyone knows who Cary Grant is, but you might catch a name or two along the way that you have never heard. At Highland Avenue, the weirdness commences. On the southeast corner is Ripley's Believe It or Not, followed by the Guinness Book of World Records Museum. On the north side is the unmistakable Hollywood Wax Museum. Should you need to see a life-size wax figure of Keanu Reeves dressed as Neo in the Matrix series, this place can scratch that itch.

Barely a block farther is Sid Grauman's first effort at an ethnically themed movie palace, the Egyptian Theatre. It is now the home of American Cinematheque, a nonprofit group dedicated to preserving film. In the next block on the north side (6667) is Musso & Frank, Hollywood's oldest eatery, featured in the remake of *Ocean's 11* and *Ed Wood*. Immediately after crossing Highland Avenue, you will see on your right the Kodak Theatre, which in 2002 became the home of the Academy Awards and is frequently used for movie premieres. Next door, the forecourt of Grauman's (now Mann's) Chinese Theatre holds the hand and foot imprints of some of the greatest stars of the cinema. The practice began with Mary Pickford and Douglas Fairbanks and continues today with such stars as Sean Connery and Meryl Streep. And while much of Hollywood can seem cheesy and prefab, the architecture and statuary of this theatre was designed by Chinese director Moon Quon and built by Chinese artisans he guided.

Just across the street is the El Capitan Theater, another example of beautiful Art Deco architecture. All Disney films are premiered here. Continue west on Hollywood Boulevard, and as you pedal you might take a moment to hum a few bars of The Kinks' classic "Hollywood Boulevard." As you approach La Brea Avenue, move into the left lane and turn as soon as you can. If you departed early enough, this shouldn't be much trouble.

Take La Brea the two blocks back to Sunset and turn right. Your course is now doubling back along your earlier route, but your view of the sights on the south side of the street should improve. You have roughly 2.75 miles back to the start of the ride.

After the Ride

No visit to Hollywood would be complete without taking some time to walk the Hollywood Walk of Fame and visit Mann's Chinese Theater.

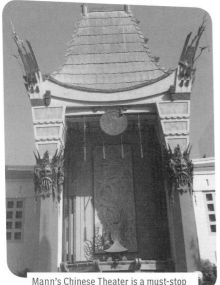

Mann's Chinese Theater is a must-stop on any tour of Hollywood.

24 The Sights of Downtown

AT A GLANCE

Length: 6 miles
Configuration: Loop
Difficulty: Easy
Climbing: 300 feet

Maximum gradient: 8%
Scenery: Historic, modern, and ethnic architecture
Exposure: Lots of shade from tall buildings
Road traffic: Heavy, except on weekend mornings
Road surface: Generally fair
Riding time: 30 minutes, 3 hours with stops
Maps: Los Angeles County *Thomas Guide* page 634

In Brief

This short circuit through downtown Los Angeles can do a lot to change one's opinion of the city. It takes in some historic and contemporary highlights of downtown LA and covers the ethnic neighborhoods of Little Tokyo and Chinatown. This route steers clear of the seedier parts of town and, if ridden on a weekend morning, avoids the treacherous downtown traffic.

Directions

From the intersection of I-10 and I-110, drive north 1.25 miles and exit at Sixth Street. Turn right at the bottom of the ramp onto Sixth and drive five blocks to South Olive Street and turn left. Turn right into the parking structure at Pershing Square.

Description

This rather novel loop has the ability to truly alter your perspective on Los Angeles. The writer Gertrude Stein famously said of Los Angeles, "There is no *there* there." Given the way the city spills over the basin, and that so few lives seem to depend on the inner workings of the cluster of high-rise offices, the perception that Los Angeles is a city without a beating heart isn't completely undeserved. What is remarkable, though, is the vibrancy of the square mile or so that can be called "downtown."

Unlike many of the rides in this guide, this one really calls for a bike lock and touring shoes or sneakers. To get the full experience, you'll need to be prepared to get off the saddle and wander around a bit.

What is now known as Los Angeles got its start back in 1771, when Father Junipero Serra founded the San Gabriel Mission. As the community grew, it was called Ciudad de Los Angeles, City of Angels. And with the signing of the Treaty of Guadalupe Hidalgo in 1848, Los Angeles and, for that matter, all of California came under the control of the United States. So while Los

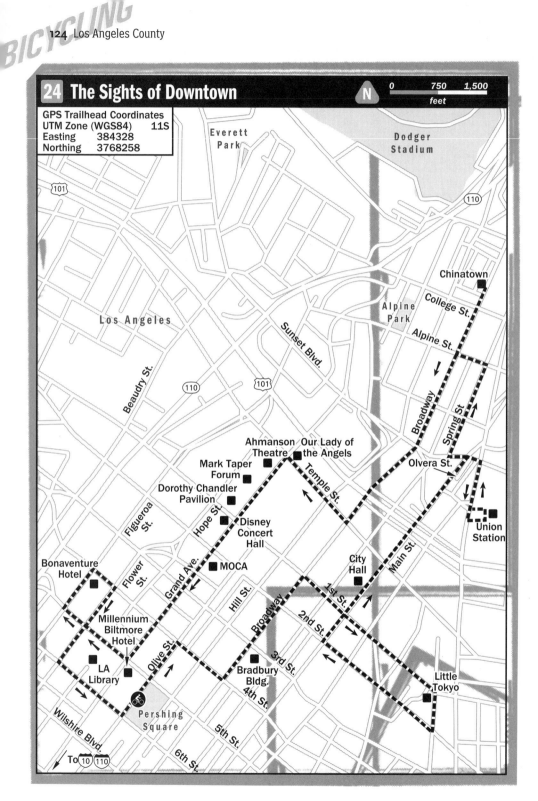

24 The Sights of Downtown

GPS Trailhead Coordinates
UTM Zone (WGS84)   11S
Easting   384328
Northing   3768258

N

0   750   1,500
feet

Everett
Park

Dodger
Stadium

101

Chinatown

Alpine
Park

College St.

Los Angeles

Sunset Blvd.

Alpine St.

Beaudry St.

110

101

Broadway

Spring St

Ahmanson Our Lady of
Theatre   the Angels

Mark Taper
Forum

Olvera St.

Dorothy Chandler
Pavilion

Temple St.

Figueroa
St.

Hope St.

Disney
Concert
Hall

Union
Station

Bonaventure
Hotel

Flower
St.

Grand Ave.

MOCA

City
Hall

Main St.

Hill St.

1st St.

Millennium
Biltmore
Hotel

Broadway

2nd St.

Olive St.

LA
Library

3rd St.

Bradbury
Bldg.

Little
Tokyo

Pershing
Square

4th St.

Wilshire Blvd

5th St.

6th St.

To 10 110

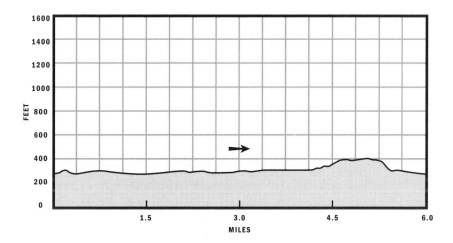

Angeles has been an "American" city for just more than 150 years, its 18th-century melting-pot roots give it a history as rich as any in the nation.

Given that this is downtown and not, say, the hills of Malibu, you may be wondering how safe it is to ride here. First, this ride doesn't go down skid row, and second, if you depart by 10 a.m. on a weekend day, traffic will be light. There will be traffic, but it will be no problem to avoid anything threatening. Easily the greatest risk on the ride will be the surface of the road itself. Be prepared for metal plates and grates, potholes, and rough surfaces.

The sights of this ride will be eerily familiar, even if you have never visited downtown before. The blockbusters filmed on these streets and in these buildings have used Los Angeles as "everywhere" in the world.

From your starting point in Pershing Square, take a moment to look at the intersection of Fifth and Hill streets at the northeast corner of the park. A beautiful Art Deco building rises there, and for those who remember the *Lou Grant* show, a spin-off

of the *Mary Tyler Moore* show, this building served as the exterior for the fictitious Los Angeles *Tribune*, where Ed Asner's character worked. To your left, across Olive Street, is the Millennium Biltmore Hotel, which will be familiar to anyone who has seen *Beverly Hills Cop, Species, The Sting, Pretty in Pink, Independence Day, True Lies,* and/or *In the Line of Fire,* among other movies. The lavish 1923 hotel has hosted a great many presidents (including John F. Kennedy), a fair number of rock stars (including The Beatles), and the 1960 Democratic National Convention.

Start by riding northeast on Olive Street, which, like many of the streets in downtown, is one-way. Cross Fifth Street and begin riding uphill to Fourth Street. This is the steepest hill you will encounter on the ride—Bunker Hill. Turn right and head downhill. Don't build up too big a head of steam because there is a light at Hill Street at the bottom of the hill. Turn left at the next intersection, at South Broadway. Pull over to the right just before the intersection with Third Street.

At your right is one of the more famous buildings in downtown, the Bradbury Building. Featured in *Chinatown, Blade Runner, Wolf* (it was the site of Jack Nicholson's office), and *Murder in the First*, among others. With its ornate ironwork and natural lighting inside (thanks to a largely glass roof), it prompted the noted architectural critic Sam Hall Kaplan to call the 1893 structure "one of the city's architectural treasures."

Continue northeast on South Broadway. As you approach Second Street, you'll see the offices of the *Los Angeles Times* to your right. With 37 Pulitzer Prizes to its credit (14 since 2000), the *LA Times* is the newspaper of record for Southern California.

Turn right at First Street and ride four blocks to Little Tokyo. On your right, you'll see the Japanese Village Plaza, with its distinctive Japanese architecture. Little Tokyo is one of three remaining Japantown communities in America. If you've ever wanted a great Japanese meal, this is the place.

Just ahead of you at the corner of East First Street and North Alameda Street is the Japanese American National Museum. Just before you reach it, turn right on South Central Avenue and immediately turn right on East Second Street. This will take you around the plaza, giving you another look at the architecture and restaurants.

Turn right on South Main Street. One of the reasons for all the right turns is that even though the streets are generally one way, making your way across four lanes of traffic to make a left turn can be a questionable proposition, even in light traffic. This way is both scenic and safer. After crossing First Street, you will pass Los Angeles City Hall, which ought to look familiar. You have seen it in the Superman television series starring George Reeves (it was the home of the *Daily Planet*), the original *The War of the Worlds* film, *Die Hard II, 48 Hours,* and plenty more.

In the next block, you pass the United States District Court building and then pass over US 101. On your right is a courtyard that begins a long, open-air market. This is Olvera Street, the birthplace of Los Angeles. The street was named for a prominent local judge in 1877 and has since been designated a historic monument. This is *the* place to be for Cinco de Mayo.

Turn right at Cesar Chavez Avenue and immediately make another right onto North Alameda Street. Move left to the turn lane and turn left at the light into the parking lot for Union Station. The location has been used in many films (*Blade Runner, Pearl Harbor, Grand Canyon, Species,* and *Dear God,* and got top billing in the eponymous *Union Station*), it is known for its Art Deco architecture and is worth walking through even if you don't plan to board a train.

Loop around the parking lot and turn right back onto North Alameda Street heading north. Turn left at Cesar Chavez Avenue, cross North Main Street, and turn right onto North Spring Street. You are now entering Chinatown. Turn left at West College Street and right on North Broadway.

The community, although no longer the center of Chinese culture in Los Angeles, dates to 1852, when Chinese immigrants were first recorded in Los Angeles. The neighborhood reached its cultural zenith, which coincided with its largest population at the turn of the century when it boasted three temples and a Chinese Opera house. Unfortunately, it was also the home to several opium dens, which led, in part, to its decline. Much of Chinatown was condemned in the following years, but it has enjoyed a resurgence and has even seen interest from Hollywood; *Rush Hour,* with Jackie Chan, is but one film that used the location. The plaza bordered by Gin Ling Way to the north and Lei Min Way to the south is well worth seeing.

Turn south on North Broadway. The street will bend slightly right and then slightly left between Cesar Chavez Avenue and US 101. After crossing the 101 and East Commercial Street, turn right on West Temple Street. Most of the last 2 miles have been rather flat, but Temple is an uphill, though not steep. Climb the two blocks to the intersection with Grand Avenue, but take a moment to notice the beautiful tile mosaic on the Hall of Records building to your left. At your right is the Cathedral of Our Lady of the Angels. Situated atop Bunker Hill, this impressive contemporary structure draws as many tourists as it does worshipers.

Turn left on Grand Avenue into the cultural heart of Los Angeles. At your right is first the Ahmanson Theater and Mark Taper Forum, followed by the Dorothy Chandler Pavilion. Upon crossing Tom Bradley Boulevard (named for the former mayor, but also known as First Street), the Frank Gehry–designed Disney Concert Hall blooms into view. The 2,265-seat hall serves as the home to the Los Angeles Philharmonic Orchestra and is an impressive and unusual sight, even for this city.

Continue south on Grand, past Second Street and the Museum of Contemporary Art (on your left) and on past Third Street. At the intersection of Fourth Street, Grand spills downhill rather suddenly and steeply. Keep your speed in check for the right turn onto Fifth Street.

After completing your right turn, you'll see the Los Angeles Central Library to your left, with its beautiful mosaic tiled roof. And to your immediate right is the 75-story Library Tower, the tallest building west of the Mississippi River and the first place vaporized in the movie *Independence Day.*

Cross Flower Street and turn right on South Figueroa Street. On your right as you approach Foutth Street is the Westin Bonaventure Hotel. Known as "The Bonaventure,"

it is likely Los Angeles's most famous hotel. With its striking mirrored facade, the hotel has appeared in some real blockbusters, among them *In the Line of Fire, True Lies, Strange Days, Ruthless People, Mr. Mom, The Poseidon Adventure,* and *Rainman.* Turn right on Fourth Street and immediately right on South Flower Street. The war-zone shootout in the film *Heat* was filmed here.

Cross Fifth Street and pass the library. The Los Angeles Marathon finishes in this block, directly in front of the library. Turn left on West Sixth Street and ride the final three blocks back to Olive Street, then turn left to return to Pershing Square.

After the Ride
The temptation to lock the bikes up and explore more of LA's great buildings will be a powerful draw. You might wait until you've had a bite to eat. There are plenty of options within walking distance of Pershing Square, but consider venturing back to Little Tokyo, Olvera Street, or Chinatown to have a truly memorable meal.

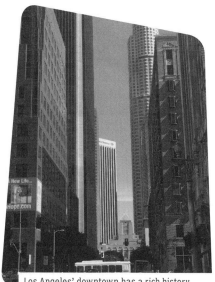

Los Angeles' downtown has a rich history with many notable buildings.

25 Fargo Street Hillclimb

AT A GLANCE

Length: 3.5 miles
Configuration: Loop
Difficulty: Difficult
Climbing: 300 feet

Maximum gradient: 33% (yes, you read that correctly)

Scenery: A beautiful park and some oddities of road building

Exposure: There is little shade on the route

Road traffic: Heavy on Glendale Boulevard but light elsewhere

Road surface: Generally good

Riding time: 30 minutes

Maps: Los Angeles County *Thomas Guide* pages 634 and 594

In Brief

The only real point to this ride is the challenge of finding out if you can ride up Fargo Street. It's the steepest street in all of Los Angeles and could easily be the steepest street in California. The ride is short, but, with so many other insanely steep streets nearby, you could easily turn this ride into an outing of masochistic achievement. Echo Park, the ride's starting point, is just to the south and is an excellent place for those with families to deposit a spouse and children and then get away for a short spin.

Directions

From the interchange of CA 110 and US 101, drive west 0.75 miles on US 101 and take Exit 4A for Glendale Boulevard. At the bottom of the ramp, turn left on Bellevue Avenue and begin looking for parking. The exit deposits you directly at Echo Park, and you should be able to find ample free parking on one of the streets around it.

Description

Much of this street's notoriety has been built through the efforts of the Los Angeles Wheelmen, one of the largest and oldest clubs in LA. Every March, the club holds a loosely organized event to see who can ride up the 0.1-mile (truly—it is less than 200 yards) hill. Given that 100 or more riders show up each year, word of the challenge has gradually spread. Certainly, the length of the hill isn't what makes it daunting: it's the grade. Maxing out at 33 percent, most folks show up at the foot of the hill and are stricken slack of jaw. The road is so steep that it is constructed of concrete; the sidewalks include steps. If you should choose to drive it, you'll see little other than sky on your way up.

The big reason to tackle the ascent when the LA Wheelmen show up isn't for the encouragement—it's for the support: they put spotters on the hill. Many riders don't make it up, which means they need to clip

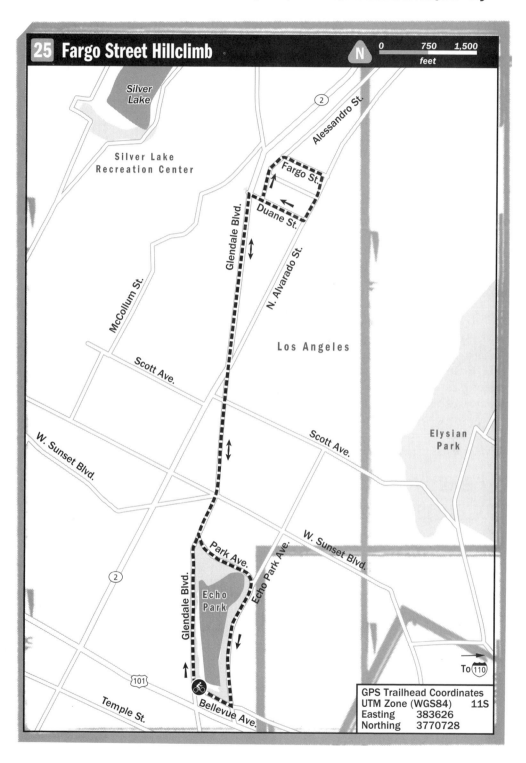

25 **Fargo Street Hillclimb**

N

0   750   1,500
feet

Silver
Lake

2

Alessandro St.

Silver Lake
Recreation Center

Fargo St.

Duane St.

Glendale Blvd.

McCollum St.

N. Alvarado St.

Los Angeles

Scott Ave.

Scott Ave.

Elysian
Park

W. Sunset Blvd.

W. Sunset Blvd.

Park Ave.

Echo Park Ave.

2

Glendale Blvd.

Echo
Park

To 110

101

Temple St.

Bellevue Ave.

GPS Trailhead Coordinates
UTM Zone (WGS84)   11S
Easting   383626
Northing   3770728

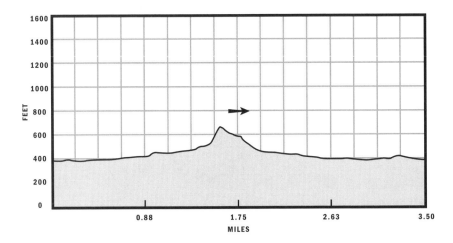

out of their pedals. It's possible to clip out before falling, but the road's incredible fall line means that the chances that you may actually arrest your motion before disaster or comedy ensue (it's a matter of perspective, really) are kinda slim. The comedy is short-lived because riders who do fall invariably slide enough to get a bit skinned up. Having

The only real point to this ride is the challenge of finding out if you can ride up Fargo Street. It's the steepest street in all of Los Angeles and could easily be the steepest street in California.

the spotters prevents raspberry picking.

To find out when the LA Wheelmen are holding their event, check their Web site (**www.lawheelmen.org**). If you choose to go on a different day, bring a friend. You two can spot each other on your ascents. And if you do bring a friend, be sure to each bring a pair of sneakers for running up the hill as you do your friendly duty.

So, how do you get up this paved cliff? Well, a truck winch is a good start. But, failing that or a crane, a triple is a good bet. A gear ratio of roughly 1-to-1 is the starting point. For road bikes it means using something on the order of 30 x 29. With a long-cage rear derailleur you can potentially turn a 32 or 34 low gear. Unless you are an especially powerful climber, compact cranks with a 34-tooth small ring are unlikely to give you the mechanical advantage necessary to prevent embarrassment.

Unlike a great many rides in this book, this ride can be attempted any time it isn't raining. Glendale Boulevard is busy during rush hour, but weekend traffic isn't so crazy that this can't be ridden in the afternoon.

To get there, begin riding north on Glendale Boulevard from the intersection of Glendale and Bellevue Avenue. Pedal just 1.3 miles before turning right onto Allesandro Street. You will see signs for the beginning of CA 2, but you turn off before it begins. Less than 300 yards from the turn, the third street on your right is Fargo. Now, for some riders, this may seem an inadequate warm-up; if that's the case for you, each of the streets to your right on your northward ride from Echo Park offers an ascent of less aggressive proportions. Be forewarned, though: As this is primarily a muscular-mechanical endeavor and not so much an aerobic one, an extended warm-up isn't really necessary.

If you make it to the top, stay on your game; the road immediately drops off steeply down to North Alvarado Street. Turn right on Alvarado and then, two blocks later, turn right on Duane Street.

With a steep pitch, little runout, no turns, fair pavement, and a rather urban setting, these downhills don't give you the chance to have much fun with gravity. So it goes. (Apologies to Kurt Vonnegut.)

Turn left back onto Glendale Boulevard. Downhill traffic on Glendale is likely your second greatest threat on this ride. Keep right while keeping an eye on the parked cars and those pulling in from side streets. Just after crossing West Sunset Boulevard, turn left on Park Avenue and make your way back to your car at Echo Park.

After the Ride

If you brought your family, there will be plenty of fun for the kids at Echo Lake, which occupies most of Echo Park. There's a small playground, plenty of ducks and geese to feed (or chase), and more. For more-adult diversions, try any of the restaurants on Sunset Boulevard, just to the north.

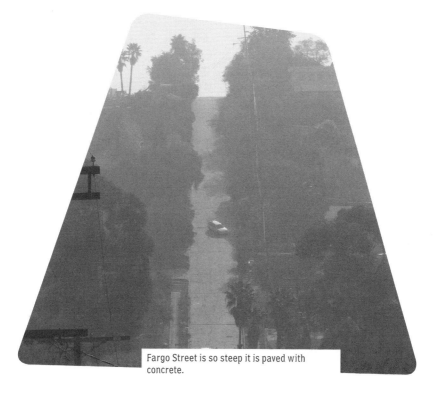

Fargo Street is so steep it is paved with concrete.

26   The Montrose Ride

AT A GLANCE

Length: 49 miles

Configuration: Loop

Difficulty: Difficult

Climbing: 1,500 feet

Maximum gradient: 7%

Scenery: Suburban neighborhoods, industrial development

Exposure: Some tree cover

Road traffic: Heavy at times

Road surface: Pretty good

Riding time: 2.5 hours

Maps: Los Angeles County *Thomas Guide*
pages 535, 565, 595, 596, 566, 597, 598, 599, 569, 568, 567, 566, and 536

In Brief

This ride takes in the San Gabriel Valley communities of La Cañada Flintridge, Pasadena, Sierra Madre, Arcadia, Monrovia, Duarte, Azusa, Covina, and Irwindale. Whereas most of the rides in this guide are designed to avoid heavy traffic, this loop takes in some well-traveled routes. The ride's claim to fame is as a group ride that has been going on for more than 20 years. If you are safely tucked into the group, these roads are much less intimidating, and the ride, which is both large and speedy, can be very enjoyable. The route itself is mostly flat at first but takes in a number of short hills near the finish.

Directions

The ride's primary start is at Descanso Gardens in La Cañada Flintridge. From the intersection of I-5 and CA 2, drive north 7.75 miles to the transition onto eastbound I-210 and exit onto Verdugo Avenue. At the bottom of the ramp, turn right and travel 0.3 miles to Descanso Drive. Turn right; there is parking on the street in front of Descanso Gardens.

Description

For roadies who like a fast group ride, the Montrose Ride is just the ticket. Peloton speeds on this ride can easily reach 35 mph. The pack for this ride is very, very large, arguably one of the largest in America. In season, its numbers can swell to 300 riders. Out of season, the ride can still see more than 150 riders. Without the group, this route isn't particularly exciting . . . or safe. With the group, the ride is much safer and more interesting.

The ride departs Descanso Gardens at 8 a.m. every Saturday. The group rolls south on Descanso Drive, which soon becomes Chevy Chase Drive, which soon becomes Berkshire Drive. None of these transitions is apparent as a turn; rather, the road

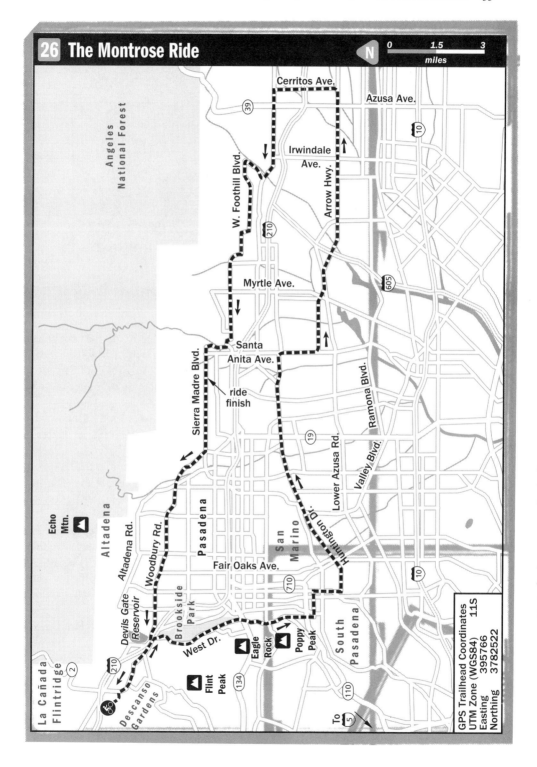

N

0   1.5   3
miles

Cerritos Ave.

Azusa Ave.

39

10

Irwindale
Ave.

W. Foothill Blvd.

Arrow Hwy.

210

Myrtle Ave.

605

Santa
Anita Ave.

Sierra Madre Blvd.

ride
finish

Ramona Blvd.

19

Lower Azusa Rd.

Valley Blvd.

Pasadena

Altadena Rd.

Woodbury Rd.

San Marino

Huntington Dr.

Echo
Mtn.

Altadena

Fair Oaks Ave.

10

Devils Gate
Reservoir

Brookside
Park

West Dr.

Eagle
Rock

Poppy
Peak

South
Pasadena

710

La Cañada
Flintridge

2

210

Flint
Peak

134

110

Descanso
Gardens

To
5

GPS Trailhead Coordinates
UTM Zone (WGS84)   11S
Easting   395766
Northing   3782522

Angeles
National Forest

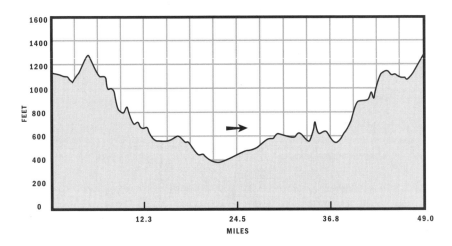

seems only to serpentine a bit. At the 2.2-mile mark, Berkshire meets Highland Drive and shifts slightly to the right. Immediately after the turn is the ride's first hill, a short kicker that you approach with such speed that a brief stomp takes you over the top. The drop down the other side is quick and precedes a sharp cut to the right where it gets yet another name change; now the road is Linda Vista Avenue.

Following the ride's first straight half-mile on Linda Vista, turn left on Salvia Canyon Road. This road drops down to

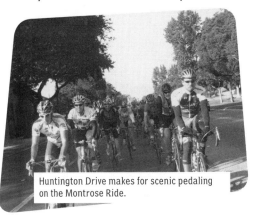

Huntington Drive makes for scenic pedaling on the Montrose Ride.

West Drive, one of the roads that encircles the Rose Bowl. At the bottom of the hill, bear right and watch not only for cars but also for pedestrians at the side of the road. Soft pedal down West 0.7 miles and turn left on Seco Drive. Immediately turn right on North Arroyo Boulevard. Arroyo climbs up a hill as it passes under CA 134. The group attacks this hill out of the saddle and in the big ring. Go full gas and stay on top of the gear as you crest the top; the downhill starts at once. Dump gear to stay tucked in.

South of CA 134, North Arroyo becomes South Arroyo. Now the fun starts. For the next 1.5 miles you fly through a very beautiful and exclusive Pasadena neighborhood. The homes are real stunners. The only trouble is, you'll never see them. The group will take this slight downhill in their 12s. Hold your line and keep pedaling through the curves. Arroyo becomes Grand Avenue and straightens but continues its downhill run.

At Mission Street in South Pasadena, turn left. Stay in the left lane as you turn; riders join you at this point, doubling the ride's size. Don't make the mistake of shifting into the small ring for the hill here. Take it in the big ring to avoid losing your place near the front of the group. The rest of the group accelerates to join. Just 0.75 miles later, turn right on Fair Oaks Avenue. A little short of a mile later, turn left on Huntington Drive. Huntington is a large, divided boulevard that, while scenic, is normally just not appropriate for cycling. You're safe in the group, but mind the stoplights. The lights come frequently, and the group doesn't run them.

Follow Huntington 6.5 miles. There is one long false flat followed by yet another downhill run. Don't downshift out of the big ring; be ready to accelerate once you crest the rise. At the 16-mile mark, to your left you will see a large commercial complex that includes a large shopping mall, the Santa Anita Park (home of the racetrack), and Methodist Hospital. Bear right on Campus Drive. One mile later, turn right on Santa Anita Drive. Another mile later, finish the last of your downhill dash by turning left on East Longden Avenue. Longden is essentially flat, but that doesn't mean you're taking it easy.

Turn left on Arrow Highway and then immediately right on Live Oak. While most of the ride up until now has been suburban and fairly upscale in its development, this region of Irwindale is essentially industrial. If it weren't for this group ride, you probably would have no reason to ride here. It's not exactly scenic, unless you have a fascination with gravel piles. Your route on Arrow Highway will climb the next 5.4 miles following the ride's lowest elevation point. The grade is the flattest of false flats, but your legs notice the difference.

Turn left at Cerritos Avenue. Your turn north marks this as your farthest point from the ride's start; the ride is not quite half over, though. Half a mile later, the ride splits at Gladstone. Those doing the shorter ride continue north, while riders

For roadies who like a fast group ride, the Montrose Ride is just the ticket.

going longer and taking in a few more hills turn right. Another half-mile up, turn left on Foothill Boulevard. Follow the group's acceleration here and swing wide to the left for the tight (beyond 90 degrees) right turn on Encanto Parkway. Coming out of the turn, downshift and make a big jump; the group accelerates here in anticipation of hitting the first of a series of hills.

Turn left on Royal Oaks Drive. This is another beyond-90-degree turn that takes many riders into the other lane. Move to the right promptly. Royal Oaks will bend left, dip 1.5 miles from the turn, then immediately bend back to the right and rise. Use the dip to generate a little speed, and maintain that momentum as you hit the rise. Turn right on Winston and pour it on. This spike of a hill is tough and requires you make a big effort to hold your place in the group. As with the other hills, don't make the mistake of downshifting into the little ring and getting dropped. Turn left on Lemon Avenue at the top and use the downhill as an opportunity to recover.

Just a little more than a half-mile later your next right turn—and hill—will be on Bradbury Road. Bradbury is a short enough, but the turn on Wildrose Avenue doesn't end the climbing, nor does the turn on Mountain Avenue, but the immediate turn onto Foothill does conclude your suffering. Ultimately, the climb is just over a half-mile, but with four turns thrown in before you have a chance to recover, it's a challenging stretch.

Following a short flat, Foothill eases into a short—2-mile—descent. Turn right on Second Avenue, immediately left on Sycamore Avenue, and right on Highland Oaks Drive. Bear left onto Elevado Avenue and make another left onto Sierra Madre Boulevard. The good news is that the climbing isn't over. Oh, wait, that's the bad news. The good news is that the climbing is almost over, and so is the hard part of the ride. Downtown Sierra Madre occupies the area around Sierra Madre and Baldwin Avenue. The group stops here for coffee roughly 100 yards after the big sprint. Chances are you'll feel grateful for the stop, if not the short runout.

The Montrose Ride doesn't finish where it starts. You're a full 15.5 miles from the start at Descanso Gardens. Fortunately, there are always some riders heading back there. You may want to hang out and have a coffee before getting back on the bike.

To get back to Descanso Gardens, begin by riding west on Sierra Madre. After 1.7 miles, turn right on New York Drive, which climbs steadily for the next 2.5 miles. At El Molino, make a brief left–right dogleg onto Woodbury Drive. At Windsor Avenue, Woodbury becomes Oak Grove Drive. The traffic here can be a little heavier because I-210 has exit and entrance ramps right here. Turn left on Berkshire Place and pass under the 210. Watch the exit ramp to your right. There is a stop sign for exiting traffic, but many cars don't come to a full stop.

The final 2 miles back to the start are all uphill. But given that you can take this at your own pace and you're on a quiet and beautiful residential street, your experience should be pretty relaxing. This is your big chance to see some of the beautiful homes of La Cañada Flintridge.

After the Ride
Take some time to visit Descanso Gardens and its incredible array of plants, especially its special collections of lilacs, roses, and camellias. The garden is home to the world's largest collection of camellias—more than 700 species—and hosts an annual camellia festival. If you're hungry, there are a number of lunch options on Verdugo Avenue near CA 2.

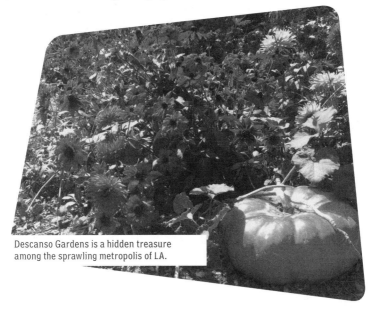

Descanso Gardens is a hidden treasure among the sprawling metropolis of LA.

27 The Rose Bowl

AT A GLANCE

Length: 3 miles
Configuration: Loop
Difficulty: Easy
Climbing: 120 feet per lap

Maximum gradient: 7%
Scenery: Arid forest, desert
Exposure: Some tree cover
Road traffic: Light
Road surface: Good
Riding time: 15 minutes
Maps: Los Angeles County *Thomas Guide* page 565

In Brief

The Pasadena Rose Bowl is known the world over as a destination for football. The Rose Bowl is as well known a bowl game as the Super Bowl; indeed, it is an older event. Today, the Tournament of Roses Parade culminates with the Rose Bowl. That wasn't always the case. In the early 20th century, the parade ended with bicycle racing. There was a track in Pasadena, and racing at the track was the crowning event. For residents of Pasadena, the Rose Bowl is more than just a football stadium. There is a golf course in the complex, and an aquatic center, too. And the roads surrounding the stadium serve as a recreation outlet for countless cyclists, skaters, joggers, and walkers. It's a lively place to spend an afternoon riding or a morning tailgating.

Directions

Travel 4.75 miles north on I-110 from the intersection of the 110 and I-5. Exit the 110 at Orange Grove Avenue. Take Orange Grove 2.4 miles north, and turn left on Rosemont Avenue. Drive north on Rosemont 0.5 miles, and turn left on Seco Street. There is parking around the stadium.

Description

As rides in this guide go, this is one of the easiest to accomplish and one of the hardest . . . to get lost on. The loop is 3 miles long and climbs in a false flat on its long, west side. There is one short hill on the long east side, and, although it is a little steeper than the false flat, it is very short.

Given the short circuit around the stadium and the golf course, this isn't the sort of loop you want to do just once, unlike the others in this book. The real point behind riding at the Rose Bowl is having the opportunity to ride with as little interference from traffic and lights as possible. And even though doing repeated laps of any course can get boring, each new lap will bring its

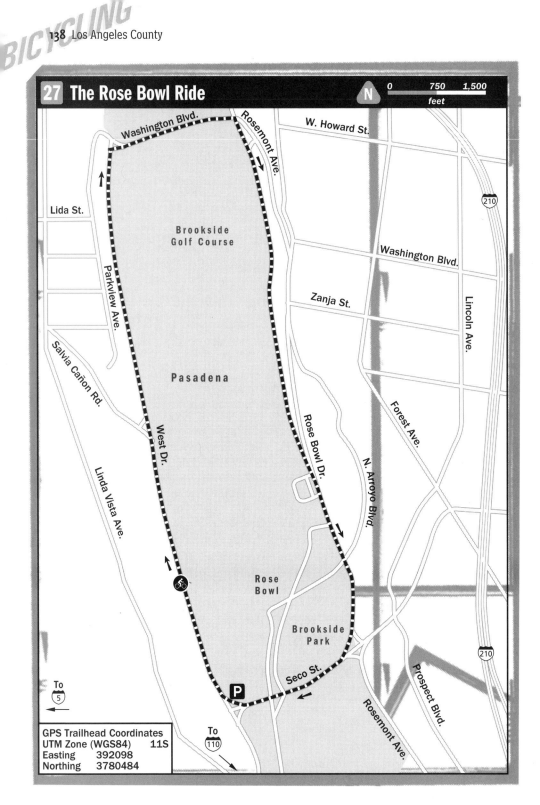

27 The Rose Bowl Ride

0   750   1,500
feet

Washington Blvd.

Rosemont Ave.

W. Howard St.

Lida St.

Brookside
Golf Course

Washington Blvd.

Zanja St.

Lincoln Ave.

Parkview Ave.

Pasadena

Salvia Cañon Rd.

West Dr.

Rose Bowl Dr.

Forest Ave.

N. Arroyo Blvd.

Linda Vista Ave.

Rose
Bowl

Brookside
Park

Prospect Blvd.

To
5

Seco St.

Rosemont Ave.

To
110

GPS Trailhead Coordinates
UTM Zone (WGS84)   11S
Easting   392098
Northing   3780484

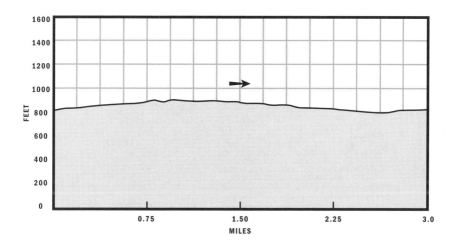

own variation to the experience.

The best way to ride the Rose Bowl is clockwise, making right turns around the grounds and therefore avoiding oncoming traffic during turns. This is how most people ride, skate, and walk or jog around. While there are always a few exceptions, this practice is ingrained for most folks. Farthest to the right are the walkers and parents with baby carriages. To their left are the joggers and skaters. Inside of them, and well into the traffic lane, is where the cyclists ride. While other rides in this guide advocate staying to the right of the shoulder, this is one ride where riding in the traffic lane is the safest, smartest thing you can do.

The directions are simple. From Seco Street at the south end of the Rose Bowl complex, ride west on Seco, turn right on West Drive, and ride north. At the first opportunity to turn right, West Washington Boulevard, turn right and take the short stretch over to Rosemont Avenue and turn right again. Riding this loop clockwise is the accepted practice. You will be safer,

and it gives cars the opportunity to enter and exit the parking lots.

Twice a week—on Tuesdays and Thursdays—during Daylight Saving Time, a group meets to ride around the Rose Bowl. They meet at 6 p.m. on the north side of Seco, the corner of Seco Street at the intersection of North Arroyo Boulevard. The real start to the ride is on West Drive, in front of the municipal golf course. The ride can be enormous at the height of the season (July and August), with more than 100 riders showing up. And with some of the LA-based pros showing up for training, the pace can be very high, with speeds reaching 26 mph on the false flat and more than 30 on the downhill. Make sure your paceline skills are sharp if you choose to ride the Rose Bowl with the group.

With only 120 feet of climbing per lap, the circuit cannot be called hilly by any means, but what you will notice after a lap or two is that the 1.3-mile stretch of West undulates a little. One mile into the incline, the road slants slightly more

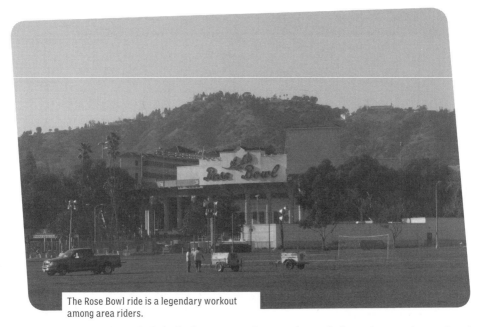

The Rose Bowl ride is a legendary workout among area riders.

upward and then dips slightly before rising as you enter the turn onto Washington Boulevard. Do not turn too sharply or you may take out a jogger. Washington loses just a bit of elevation before taking you into the next turn, which will give your pedal stoke a boost.

The run south on Rosemont Avenue is a rollicking affair. Stick it in the big ring for the 100-foot drop over the next 1.1 miles. It's not a downhill, per se, but it loses just enough elevation to make you feel like you can achieve car-like speeds on a flat. Inspiration of that sort can make for great training. There is one bump of a rise just as you pass the south end of the stadium; hit it out of the saddle and power through to the turn on Seco. The road will continue to drop on Seco for the next 0.3 miles, and then you get a noticeable rise, bringing you into the turn back onto West. When you started, the rise wasn't apparent, but when you hit it at speed, you'll see how it robs you of momentum. The question is,

do you downshift or do you dig in for the longer effort?

After the Ride

With downtown Pasadena just a mile southeast, a visit to its selection of shops and restaurants is a must. From microbrewed beers to sophisticated French cuisine, you can find anything you are looking for in Old Town Pasadena.

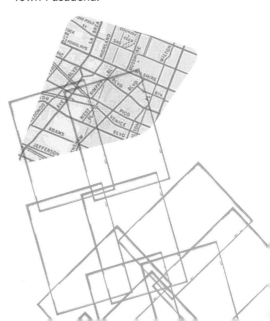

28 San Marino Loop

AT A GLANCE

Length: 8.5 miles
Configuration: Loop
Difficulty: Easy
Climbing: Less than 200 feet

Maximum gradient: 6%

Scenery: Stately homes, stunning gardens

Exposure: Not much because of the number of large trees

Road traffic: Mostly light

Road surface: Good to excellent

Riding time: 45 minutes

Maps: Los Angeles County *Thomas Guide* pages 596 and 566

In Brief

The San Marino Loop is a short and easy ride through one of Southern California's most beautiful communities. This is a home tour, plain and simple. What's different about this is that it takes you by some truly stately manses, where seemingly every front yard is a garden. The ride also circumnavigates the Huntington Library and Gardens.

Directions

From the intersection of I-10 and I-110, drive north on I-110 into Pasadena. Exit I-110 at Fair Oaks Avenue and turn right. At Mission Street, turn left and take it 1 mile to South Los Robles Avenue. Turn left at Monterey Road and take it to Virginia Road. You can park in the parking lot of Lacy Park or on the street nearby.

Description

In a metropolis with some of the most afflu-

ent ZIP codes in the entire country, San Marino is where the Carnegies, Vanderbilts, and Rockefellers would have lived, had they settled in Southern California. This is a community where the homes have the appearance of old money, even if the property turned over just last year.

Interestingly, the community isn't terribly old. It was founded in 1926, and its first mayor was George Patton Sr., the father of the famed general George Patton Jr.

This ride features a number of turns, but, because this is an entirely residential neighborhood, the course relies on mostly right turns and the few left turns across traffic happen in more secluded spots.

To begin, head south on Virginia Road, past Lacy Park. The park is a popular local recreation spot and features a paved loop where cyclists can ride. This loop is a great ride for a family with small children.

Turn right on Monterey Street. This is a fairly large avenue with a wide shoulder.

BICYCLING

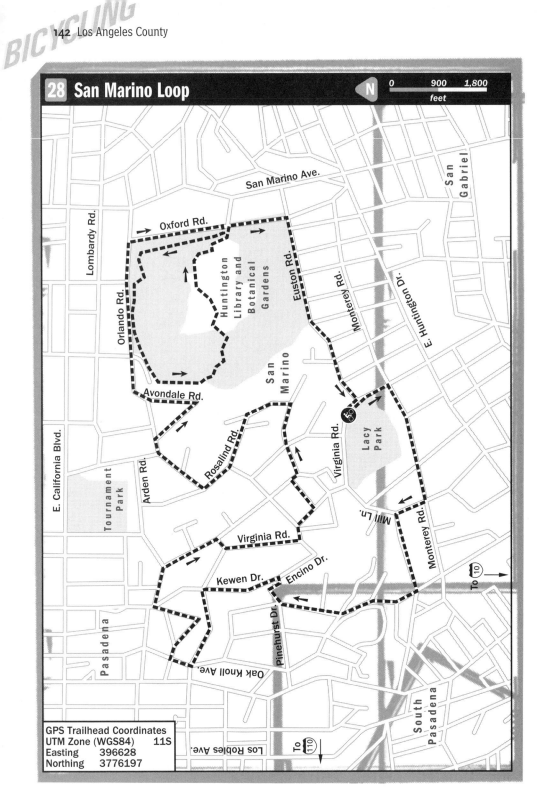

N

| 0 | 900 | 1,800 |

feet

San Marino Ave.

Lombardy Rd.

Oxford Rd.

Euston Rd.

San Gabriel

Monterey Rd.

E. Huntington Dr.

Orlando Rd.

Huntington Library and Botanical Gardens

San Marino

Avondale Rd.

Rosalind Rd.

Virginia Rd.

Lacy Park

E. California Blvd.

Tournament Park

Arden Rd.

Virginia Rd.

Mill Ln.

Monterey Rd.

To 10

Kewen Dr.

Encino Dr.

Pinehurst Dr.

Oak Knoll Ave.

Pasadena

South Pasadena

Los Robles Ave.

To 110

GPS Trailhead Coordinates
UTM Zone (WGS84)   11S
Easting   396628
Northing   3776197

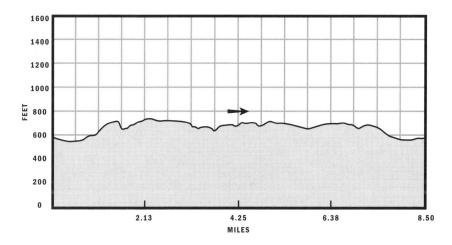

Traffic is fairly light here.

Turn right on Old Mill Road. The road begins to climb then bends left before intersecting with Oak Knoll Avenue. Turn right on Oak Knoll, which will continue to climb. This is the only significant uphill of the entire ride. The 0.8-mile uphill climbs just more than 200 feet for a 4-percent grade.

At the next real intersection, turn right on Hillcrest Avenue. The intersection features a rather odd fork, and Hillcrest bears right at about a 45-degree angle. The road continues to climb for another 100 yards. The homes in this area embody stately grandeur and are impressive for both their size and architectural flourishes.

Turn right on Pinehurst Avenue. The road turns to the right and heads downhill between two homes. Where Pinehurst intersects Kewen Drive turn left and begin following the road up the slight hill.

The homes on Kewen are almost uniformly shrouded in foliage. The temperature in this depression is generally at least 5°F cooler than in the surrounding area. In addition to trees, the front yards of almost all the homes in this stretch have gardens. From stands of bamboo to riots of perennial color, the area is truly an oasis.

Kewen intersects Oak Knoll and Fairfield Circle. Oak Knoll is a little busier here; make a quick right on Fairfield Circle and follow the loop around the 200 yards of manicured lawns. When Fairfield rejoins Oak Knoll Circle, turn right on Oak Knoll and make an immediate right onto Arden Drive.

The very next right turn is on Oak Grove Avenue. Just 0.2 miles farther, turn right on Virginia Road for a half-mile downhill. It's easy to overshoot the left onto Mesa Road. If you do, don't worry. There is a bridge overgrown with foliage; if you pass beneath it, you'll know you rode too far.

Following your left turn, there is a dog-leg to the right onto Oak Grove Avenue. Initially, the road is flat, but it quickly curves right and dips briefly but steeply. Take care on the downhill and the following uphill.

Turn right onto Rosalind Road; the road rises slightly. Downshift a cog and turn right onto Orlando Road. Orlando runs along the northern edge of Huntington Library and

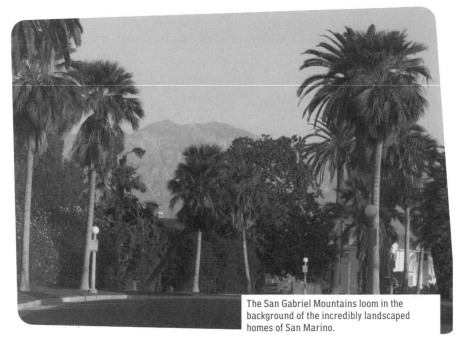

The San Gabriel Mountains loom in the background of the incredibly landscaped homes of San Marino.

Gardens. Huntington Library is known for its extraordinary collection of rare books. It continues to be one of the most extensively used research libraries in the United States, thanks in part to the presence of such gems as a Gutenberg Bible, the first two quartos of *Hamlet,* and the first seven drafts of Henry David Thoreau's *Walden.*

Follow Orlando along the northern edge of the gardens. Turn right on Oxford Street, and 0.3 miles down make another right into the Huntington's gardens. You enter on North Bound Drive, which quickly bends left and becomes West Bound Drive before becoming Director's Drive, which bends left and takes you south to the library as North Canyon Road. Traverse the road in front of the library and then join East Bound Drive to exit the grounds. This should give you just enough of a taste to inspire your return after the ride.

Turn right back onto Oxford Road and take it downhill to Euston Road, then turn right. From here you have a 0.7-mile return on Euston Road to Virginia Road and your car.

For families with young children, Lacy Park presents an excellent opportunity for the whole family to ride together: inside the park is a short loop where families can ride with small children and no fear of traffic.

After the Ride

Plenty of great restaurants can be found in nearby South Pasadena. Near the intersection of California Boulevard and Lake, there's quite a selection. But before you go, at least take an hour to tour the Huntington Library and Gardens. Man's ability to preserve beauty shows well here.

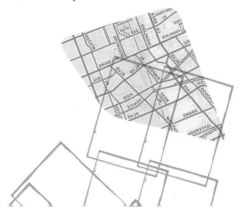

29 Turnbull Canyon Loop

AT A GLANCE

Length: 23 miles

Configuration: Loop

Difficulty: Moderate

Climbing: 2,000 feet

Maximum gradient: 8%

Scenery: Some stunning expanses of bougainvillea, views of the San Gabriel Valley and wooded canyon land

Exposure: Mornings and late afternoons can be overcast

Road traffic: Moderate

Road surface: Good

Riding time: 2.5 hours

Maps: Los Angeles County *Thomas Guide* pages 678, 708, 707, and 677

In Brief

This central Los Angeles route takes in some surprisingly fun terrain hidden within the sprawling metropolis. Turnbull Canyon is arguably the biggest climb between the San Gabriel Mountains and the Palos Verdes Peninsula.

Directions

From the intersection of I-605 and CA 60, travel east on the 60. Exit at Azusa Avenue and turn right. At Colima Road, turn left and immediately turn right into the parking lot for Schabarum Park.

Description

Exit the parking lot and turn right on Colima Road. This area is a highly developed commercial corridor. Across the street is the Puente Hills Mall; traffic here can be fairly heavy at times. This ride is best accomplished early on weekend mornings or after rush hour on weekday mornings.

After just more than a mile on Colima, the road will begin to rise slightly; turn right on Larkvane Road. This road will take you into a residential area and allow you to avoid another commercial development. Larkvane intersects Crosshaven Drive. Turn left and immediately turn right on Fullerton Road. While it is a large avenue, Fullerton has a wide shoulder and isn't as heavily traveled as Colima.

Your next turn will come 1.2 miles later, as you climb a very gradual rise. Fullerton will turn to the right; the road that continues straight becomes Harbor Boulevard. Fullerton continues to climb and winds through a quieter residential development. After climbing another 0.8 miles, Fullerton intersects East Road. East is a smaller two-lane road through a surprisingly quiet neighborhood featuring truly fun terrain. Turn right on East and begin descending. The road descends a half-mile before beginning a series of three short hills. The fun of

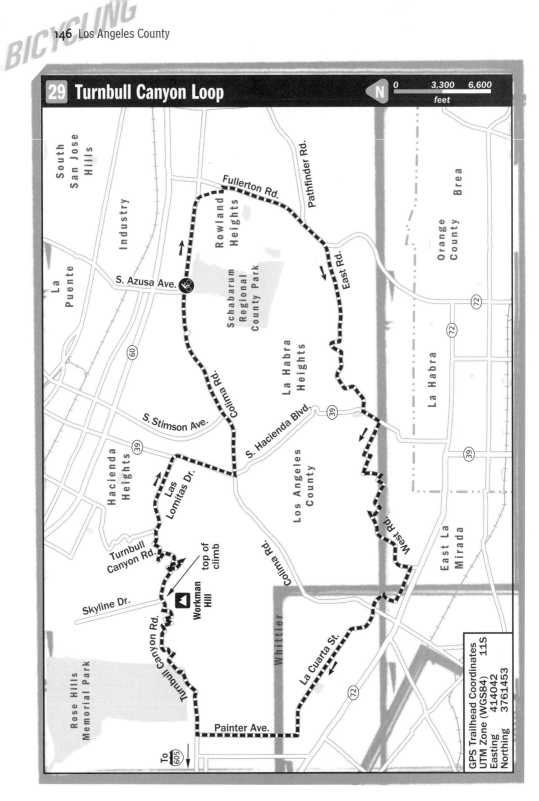

29 Turnbull Canyon Loop

N

| 0 | 3,300 | 6,600 |

feet

South San Jose Hills

Industry

La Puente

Fullerton Rd.

Pathfinder Rd.

Rowland Heights

Orange County

Brea

S. Azusa Ave.

Schabarum Regional County Park

East Rd.

La Habra Heights

72

72

60

Colima Rd.

S. Stimson Ave.

S. Hacienda Blvd.

39

La Habra

39

Hacienda Heights

39

Las Lomitas Dr.

Los Angeles County

Turnbull Canyon Rd.

top of climb

Colima Rd.

West Rd.

East La Mirada

Skyline Dr.

Workman Hill

Turnbull Canyon Rd.

Whittier

La Cuarta St.

72

Rose Hills Memorial Park

Painter Ave.

To 605

GPS Trailhead Coordinates
UTM Zone (WGS84)   11S
Easting   414042
Northing   3761453

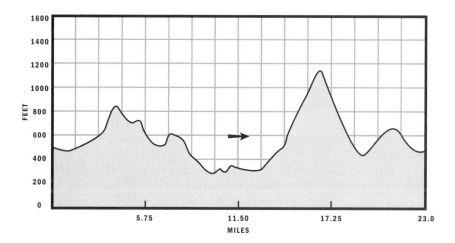

this section is to try to maintain as much speed as possible through the descent and turns so that you can attack the hills in the big ring. It's a rollicking good time.

Following the third hill, you encounter a stoplight at Hacienda Boulevard. Turn left and descend 0.25 miles to West Road; turn right. West offers the same features as East Road: a serpentine route through a quiet residential area with three short hills to power over. A final runout will take you toward Whittier Boulevard. You'll see the large commercial development ahead. Just before reaching the large thoroughfare, turn right on Janine Drive. This will allow you to avoid the traffic on Whittier. A few blocks later, Janine intersects La Serna Drive. Turn right on La Serna and begin climbing a short hill. Turn left at your next opportunity (roughly 0.25 miles farther) onto Carretera Drive. Cross Colima Road, and two blocks later turn right on La Cuarta Street. You will continue through a residential neighborhood on La Cuarta for nearly 2 miles.

At Painter Avenue, turn right. Painter is a false flat that climbs 1.4 miles to Beverly Boulevard. It does kick up a bit just before you turn right onto Beverly. A quarter-mile after that turn, the road becomes Turnbull Canyon Road. Including the rise up Painter, the ascent gains 900 feet in 4.2 miles for an average gradient of 4 percent. The 680-foot climb up Turnbull itself is 2.4 miles with an average gradient of a little more than 5 percent. The grade actually starts gently, gradually getting steeper as you gain altitude. It is an excellent road to train on for climbing power. And with 16 distinct turns and switchbacks, your views are

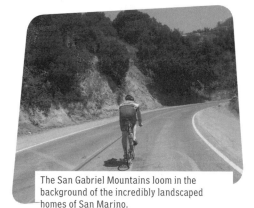

The San Gabriel Mountains loom in the background of the incredibly landscaped homes of San Marino.

ever-changing; for most of the climb, you can't even see the top. Without a firm sense of your distance to the top (unless you have done it enough to have memorized the turns), this is a climb where it's easy to overextend yourself and blow a turn or two from the top.

Once you summit, pull off to the left onto Skyline Drive. After finishing the climb, you deserve an opportunity to catch your breath and have a bite to eat. Your view of the canyon—surprisingly wild terrain, given your situation in central Los Angeles—imparts a great sense of accomplishment.

The ensuing descent is fun, if a little technical. Roll out east on Turnbull Canyon. The roller-coaster ride will drop 550 feet in 1.7 miles with just as many twists and turns on the way down as you encountered on the way up, but there are only three switchbacks that really require caution. It is common to catch traffic on the way down; a bicycle can descend these roads much faster than most cars can.

This central Los Angeles route takes in some surprisingly fun terrain hidden within the sprawling metropolis. Turnbull Canyon is arguably the biggest climb between the San Gabriel Mountains and the Palos Verdes Peninsula.

At the intersection with Las Lomitas Drive, Turnbull Canyon bends to the left. Go straight through the stop sign onto Las Lomitas. At the next intersection, turn right onto Tetley Street. Las Lomitas and Tetley continue to scrub altitude, making the pedaling easy. Following a brief rise, turn right on South Hacienda Boulevard. Hacienda is a large road with a sizable shoulder. The good news is that you will be on Hacienda less than a mile. As you approach Colima Road, move into the left turn lane. Commercial development here means there is a fair amount of traffic at all but the earliest hours.

After turning onto Colima, you encounter the final rise of the ride. A short dig gets you over the hump and to the final downhill run back to Schabarum Park. Colima has a bike lane to the right, and the lanes are wide, so despite the traffic, you should feel safe as you return to the park. The entrance to Schabarum Park comes immediately after you cross Azusa Avenue; turn right into the parking lot.

After the Ride
Schabarum Park sits across the street from the Puente Hills Mall. Aside from the usual collection of stores and shops, the mall has a number of restaurants ranging from fast food to more traditional sit-down restaurants. There are a number of other restaurants in the area.

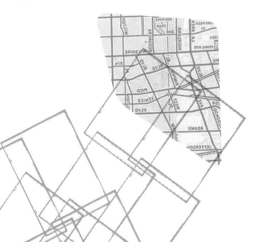

30 Santa Fe Dam Loop

AT A GLANCE

Length: 25 miles
Configuration: Loop
Difficulty: Moderate
Climbing: 350 feet
Maximum gradient: 9%
Scenery: Two rivers, heavy industry, and a large quarry
Exposure: There is really no shade except at Santa Fe Dam Recreation Area
Road traffic: Moderate
Road surface: Fair to good
Riding time: 2 hours
Maps: Los Angeles County *Thomas Guide* pages 636, 637, 597, and 598

In Brief

This loop through Rosemead, Arcadia, and El Monte gives cyclists a peaceful loop ride in an area better known for heavy industry than scenic cycling. The loop begins by heading northbound on the upper Rio Hondo Bike Path. Following a short section of road, there is a ride along the Santa Fe Dam Bike Path and then a return on the upper San Gabriel Bike Path. There is little climbing on the route; the bike path climbs gently on the way out and descends on the return.

Directions

From the intersection of CA 60 and I-710, drive east on the 60 and exit at Rosemead Boulevard. Drive 0.5 miles north on Rosemead to the entrance to the Whittier Narrows Dam Recreation Area. Once inside the park, turn left and look for parking.

Description

The entrance to the Rio Hondo Bike Path is at the southwest corner of the park. Ride up the ramp to the path, which will parallel CA 60. The first turn comes barely 0.3 miles along the path. Turn right to begin following the path north. Whittier Narrows Recreation Area offers a great many recreation options for nearby residents. As you ride north, you will first pass a model-airplane flying area; immediately following that is a rifle range (one wonders what happens if a model plane strays too far north).

Over the next 6 miles, the bike path climbs just more than 100 feet; that makes for a less-than-1-percent grade. To your left is the Rio Hondo River, which, because of development in Los Angeles, looks more like a spillway than a natural body of water.

At the 4-mile mark, you reach the El Monte Airport. This is a small-aircraft airport with a single runway paralleling the bike path. The airport serves as a training site for a variety of aeronautic students, including helicopter pilots. Watch for

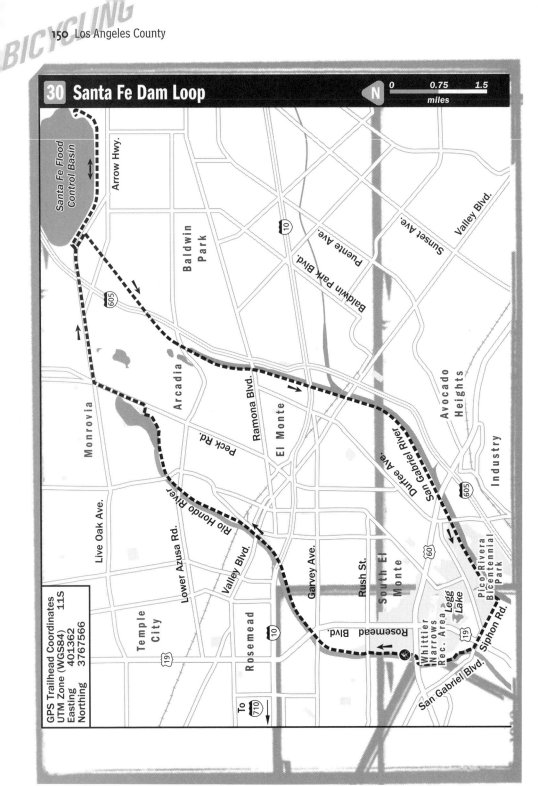

N

0   0.75   1.5
miles

Santa Fe Flood Control Basin

Arrow Hwy.

Baldwin Park

605

10

Puente Ave.

Baldwin Park Blvd.

Sunset Ave.

Valley Blvd.

Arcadia

Monrovia

Ramona Blvd.

El Monte

Avocado Heights

Industry

605

Peck Rd.

Live Oak Ave.

Rio Hondo River

Durfee Ave.

San Gabriel River

Lower Azusa Rd.

Valley Blvd.

Garvey Ave.

Rush St.

South El Monte

60

Pico Rivera

Bicentennial Park

Temple City

Rosemead

10

19

Rosemead Blvd.

Whittier Narrows Rec. Area

Legg Lake

19

Siphon Rd.

San Gabriel Blvd.

To 710

GPS Trailhead Coordinates
UTM Zone (WGS84)   11S
Easting   401362
Northing   3767566

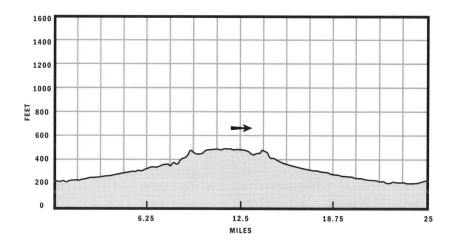

helicopters doing touch-and-gos as you pass.

Another 2 miles on, you reach a small lake and the end of the bike path. Pass through the parking lot and follow the driveway to Peck Road. Turn left onto Peck and follow it north to Live Oak Avenue; turn right. Ride 1.8 miles on Live Oak and watch for the parking area at the entrance to the bike path up onto the Santa Fe Dam.

You'll see an entrance to the bike path at your left. Move to the left of the lane and turn onto the ramp up to the path. Just 100 yards up the path, turn right to ride up to the top of the dam. This hill is rather steep, reaching a 9-percent grade before topping out. Once on top, you'll find views of the surrounding area are generally limited only by air quality. As this area is within the San Gabriel Valley, which isn't actually known for crystal-clear air, visibility can be fewer than 10 miles.

The bike path atop the Santa Fe Dam is 2.1 miles long. Views to the north take in the park below and the San Gabriel Mountains, which rise just a few miles away. Views to the south aren't the most interesting. Irwindale is perhaps best known for its speedway, but much of the development here is industrial and includes an electrical substation and a quarry.

From the dam, ride down into the park. The flood-control basin includes a man-made lake. It's a great spot for a picnic, or, at the very least, a good spot to stop for a drink and a snack. There are restrooms here as well.

The ride back up the dam isn't terribly steep. Once at the other end, be careful

The bike path atop Santa Fe Dam makes for great protected riding with an unobstructed vista.

on the rather steep descent; it's easy to exceed 30 mph on the descent, but there isn't much runout. Brake firmly as you near the bottom, and turn left to head back out to the parking area. Pass the entrance you used to join the bike path, and continue another 50 yards. Cross the street and enter the upper San Gabriel River Bike Path.

This next leg of the ride, on the San Gabriel River Bike Path, will see you lose all the elevation gained thus far. The difference between the San Gabriel River Bike Path and the Rio Hondo River Bike Path is that Rio Hondo is graded over a very slight incline, whereas the San Gabriel can run utterly flat for 100 yards or more followed by sharp grades. Because of the intermittent inclines (or declines, depending on your direction), this path can make for a very fun workout. Use the downhills to accelerate; the battle is to maintain your speed until the next downhill. By the time you reach the sharp right turn in the path, you'll be pretty worked. The turn comes at 22.5 miles; go past the left that allows riders to continue south on the San Gabriel River Bike Path.

The path ends at the intersection of Rosemead Boulevard and Durfee Avenue, but just before you reach the intersection there is an opportunity to cross Durfee. Pass through the chain-link fence and turn left on Durfee. Cross Rosemead and, less than 100 yards later, ride up the ramp and enter the upper Rio Hondo Bike Path. Pass through the chain-link fence and continue north on the path.

Depending on the time of year you do the ride, the foliage here can be surprisingly thick. The path bends right 0.9 miles after you enter from the road. From here it is less than a half-mile straight back to the park.

After the Ride

You might consider spending a little time watching the model airplanes fly before leaving the park. The nearest dining options are at the Montebello Town Center. To get there, drive south on Rosemead, turn right on San Gabriel Boulevard, and then turn left on Town Center Drive.

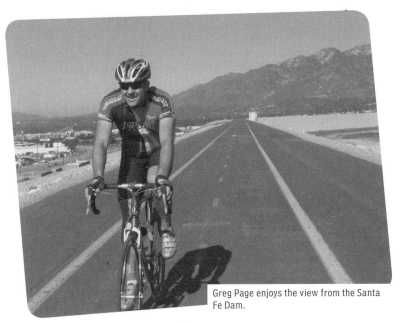

Greg Page enjoys the view from the Santa Fe Dam.

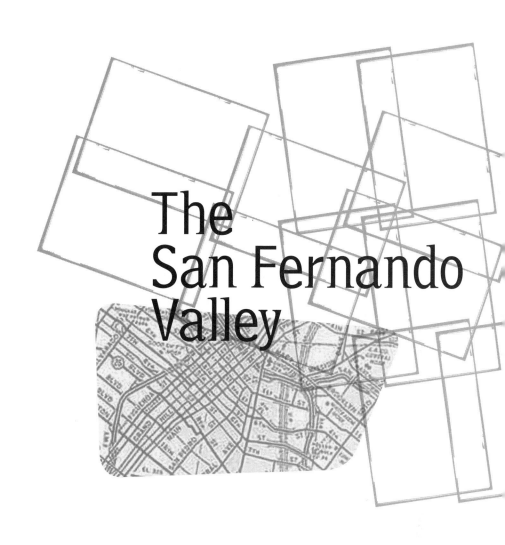

The
San Fernando
Valley

31 Sepulveda Dam Recreation Area Bike Path

AT A GLANCE

Length: 7.5 miles
Configuration: Loop
Difficulty: Easy
Climbing: Less than 100 feet
Maximum gradient: 2%
Scenery: Arid forest, desert
Exposure: Occasional shade from trees lining the bike path
Road traffic: None
Road surface: Good
Riding time: 30 minutes
Maps: Los Angeles County *Thomas Guide* pages 561 and 531

In Brief

The Sepulveda Dam Recreation Area is a multiuse park encompassing more than 2,000 acres around the dam of the Los Angeles River. Recreation facilities include a lake, an archery range, two golf courses, tennis courts, a model-airplane flying area, and one of LA's two velodromes. The bike path circles the main body of the park, giving you an opportunity to view other people enjoying themselves. This is a very popular bike path, and you are likely to see other riders no matter what time of day you visit. The ride features no steep or sustained hills. Should you need to rent bicycles or skates, there is a place to do so near the parking area.

Directions

From the interchange of CA 101 and I-405, drive 2 miles west on the 101 and exit at Balboa Boulevard. At the bottom of the ramp, turn right and drive north 0.75 miles, then turn right into the driveway for the Sepulveda Dam Recreation Area. Follow the road around to the east side of Balboa Lake; there you will find plenty of free parking and an easy entrance to the bike path.

Description

From the parking area at Balboa Lake, ride east and turn right onto the bike path to head south. The path's meandering route carves a lazy serpentine through the parkland. Given the encroaching metropolis, this recreation spot is a welcome haven. This early leg of the ride offers good but not great views of the lake, from which you are separated by the access road. However, the views of the trees around you make up for that because they hide the nearby commercial development.

The path will guide you west, over a bridge above part of the Los Angeles River and on toward Balboa Boulevard. At Balboa, the path will pass beneath the

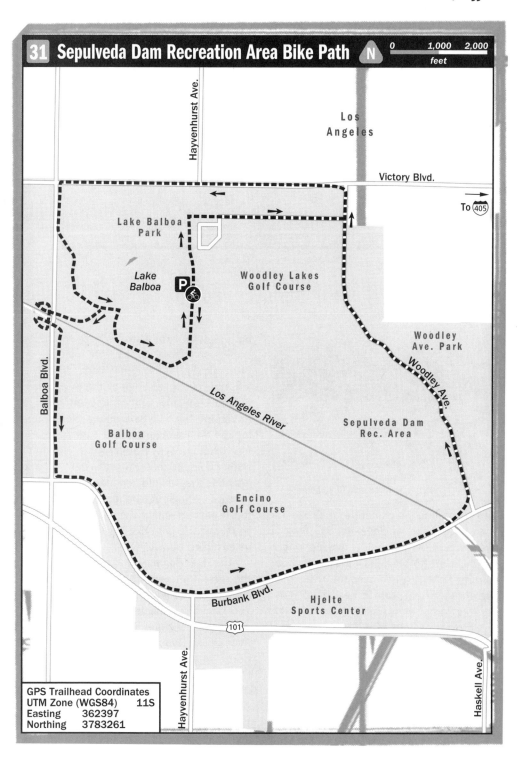

31 Sepulveda Dam Recreation Area Bike Path

N

0   1,000   2,000
feet

Hayvenhurst Ave.

Los
Angeles

Victory Blvd.

To 405

Lake Balboa
Park

Lake
Balboa

P

Woodley Lakes
Golf Course

Woodley
Ave. Park

Woodley Ave.

Balboa Blvd.

Los Angeles River

Balboa
Golf Course

Sepulveda Dam
Rec. Area

Encino
Golf Course

Burbank Blvd.

Hjelte
Sports Center

101

Hayvenhurst Ave.

Haskell Ave.

GPS Trailhead Coordinates
UTM Zone (WGS84)   11S
Easting   362397
Northing   3783261

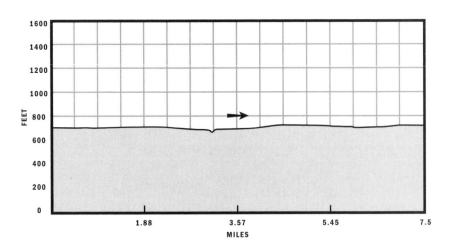

be grateful for the path because the heavy traffic isn't likely to be too inviting. At Burbank Boulevard, the path will turn left and follow the edge of the park to the Balboa Municipal Golf Course entrance. At this point, the bike path enters the parking lot and the route gets a little funny. Parking has been moved around a bit, so don't bother trying to follow the bike path's markers here; they are old and inaccurate. Watch for cars pulling out, and just make your way to the eastern end of the parking lot, where you'll see the path exit the lot and resume its eastward trajectory.

The bike path will continue to edge the recreation area. To your left is the golf course, and to your right Burbank Avenue. You could say the left half of your route is scenic. Continue 1.4 miles to Woodley Avenue. At Woodley, turn left and head north on the path. Because Woodley cuts through the recreation area, you will find that the noise and traffic drop tremendously as you ride away from Burbank. The 1.2-mile stretch of path rises slightly on this leg, gaining about 40 feet of elevation, not

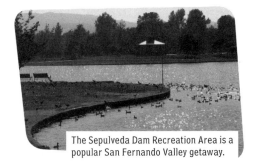

The Sepulveda Dam Recreation Area is a popular San Fernando Valley getaway.

boulevard. You'll cross under the road and then trace a sort of cloverleaf by riding up the ramp on the other side, making a right-hand U-turn (to head back toward Balboa), turning right to pass over the river, making another right turn to head back down another ramp, and, finally, making a right U-turn to pass beneath Balboa once again. Back on the east side of Balboa, but now on the south bank of the Los Angeles River, make one final right-hand U-turn and then immediately make a left to head south on the bike path. Again, kinda convoluted, but also kinda fun in a quirky sort of way.

The course parallels Balboa, and you'll

really enough to slow you down much.

As you head north toward Woodley Park and Apollo 11 Model Airplane Field, you'll begin to hear what sounds like a weed eater on steroids. If you recall the line-control planes from years ago, you'll note that what you see to your left is substantially different from them. These "models" are surprisingly sophisticated. You may see prop-driven acrobatic planes, helicopters, and even model jets. Yes, jets. These are real working jet engines that sound like Chihuahua-sized F-18s.

North of Woodley Park is an access road for one of the golf courses. Should you wish to make a quick return to your car or avoid the noise of the traffic north of you on Victory Boulevard, turn left and take the access road a half-mile to reach the left turn back onto the bike path. The parking lot is just 0.25 miles south.

If you choose to continue, you will encounter a crossing another 100 yards north. There are special bus routes in this part of Los Angeles. This one features its own road, which parallels Victory Boulevard. Watch for the crossing signal. The buses barrel through here fast to make the journey to downtown as quickly as possible. Don't end up in an accident report.

At Victory Boulevard, the path turns left and winds through trees and manicured landscaping for a mile, bringing you back to Balboa. Be careful as you approach Balboa, though. Oddly, there is an office building on the corner, so watch for cars entering and exiting its parking lot from Victory. At the corner, turn left, watch for traffic at the other entrance, and then stop and wait for the crossing signal at the bus route.

Your route south will cut inland and away from Balboa just 0.2 miles from the corner. As you pedal back into the oasis, the noise will drop and, after you crest a small rise in the park, you'll gain a view of the lake once again.

Cross the access road and rejoin the path you rode earlier; turn left to return to the parking lot. Or, to take another loop, turn right after crossing the road.

The Sepulveda Dam Recreation Area is a multiuse park encompassing more than 2,000 acres around the dam of the Los Angeles River.

After the Ride

The San Fernando Valley is full of dining and shopping opportunities. There are a great many good restaurants on Burbank Boulevard at which you might have a post-ride meal. Before you leave the park, enjoy the lake a bit and take in all the waterfowl there. You might consider taking the access road back to Woodley and driving down to Apollo 11 Field to spend a few minutes watching the model airplanes fly. They're fascinating contraptions, and some of the pilots display truly impressive skills.

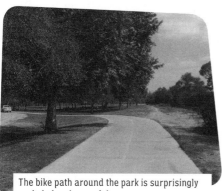

The bike path around the park is surprisingly secluded and peaceful.

32 Sherman Oaks Loop

AT A GLANCE

Length: 16 miles

Configuration: Loop

Difficulty: Moderate (provided you have low gears)

Climbing: 1,600 feet

Maximum gradient: 18%

Scenery: Impressive homes, sweeping views of the valley and the vertiginous canyons

Exposure: Some occasional shade from trees

Road traffic: Light to moderate

Road surface: Generally good

Riding time: 2 hours

Maps: Los Angeles County *Thomas Guide* pages 562, 561, and 591

In Brief

Taking in the north side of the Santa Monica Mountains, this ride traverses roads in the swanky community of Sherman Oaks (though the first climb is technically in Encino). Views here are of homes that each benefited from the hand of an individual architect rather than the cookie-cutter stamp of a developer. The ride also boasts the steepest climb of more than a half-mile in LA County, Calneva Drive, which makes for an excellent challenge early in the ride.

Directions

From the interchange of I-405 and US 101, drive 2 miles east on the 101 and exit at Woodman Avenue. At the bottom of the ramp, turn right on Woodman and drive 0.5 miles to Ventura Boulevard. Turn right and begin looking for street parking. There is plenty of metered parking here. Free parking can be found on the residential streets nearby.

Description

Sherman Oaks would be the nicest suburb in a great many cities in America. Unfortunately, it suffers in the shadow of a great many top-shelf communities, including Beverly Hills and Santa Monica. Shrouded by the north face of the Santa Monica Mountains, views here are good on hazy days and spectacular on clear days. And while the San Fernando Valley may not seem like the first choice of Hollywood celebrities, a great many celebs and otherwise-successful folks have built a personal paradise above the canyon roads.

This ride is built around two significant, roughly-2-mile climbs. The first starts pleasantly enough. But with a little more than a half-mile to go, it turns steeply upward. If your bike is sufficiently low-geared—as in you possess a triple or a compact with a 25- or 27-tooth rear cog—you'll be fine. If, however, your bike is equipped with a more traditional 39-tooth small ring, you are in for an adventure. Now, if your first name is

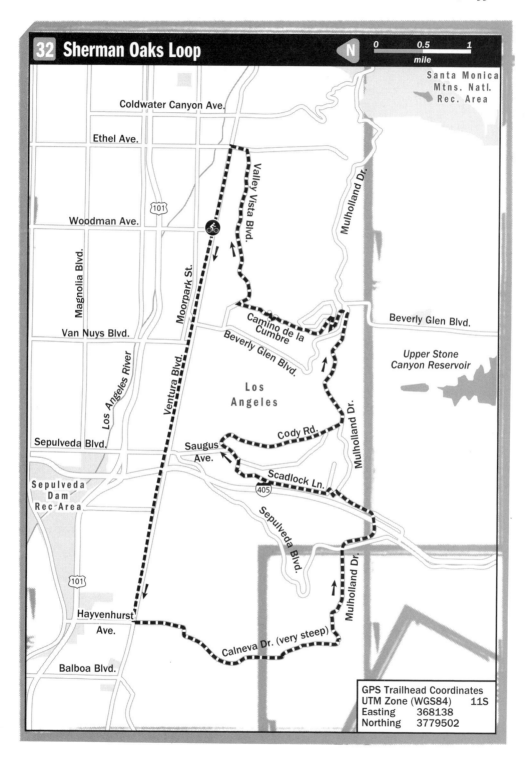

Coldwater Canyon Ave.

Santa Monica
Mtns. Natl.
Rec. Area

Ethel Ave.

Valley Vista Blvd.

Mulholland Dr.

101

Woodman Ave.

Magnolia Blvd.

Van Nuys Blvd.

Camino de la
Cumbre

Beverly Glen Blvd.

Beverly Glen Blvd.

Upper Stone
Canyon Reservoir

Moorpark St.

Los Angeles River

Ventura Blvd.

Los
Angeles

Cody Rd.

Mulholland Dr.

Sepulveda Blvd.

Saugus
Ave.

Scadlock Ln.

405

Sepulveda
Dam
Rec Area

Sepulveda Blvd.

Mulholland Dr.

101

Hayvenhurst
Ave.

Calneva Dr. (very steep)

Mulholland Dr.

Balboa Blvd.

GPS Trailhead Coordinates
UTM Zone (WGS84)   11S
Easting   368138
Northing   3779502

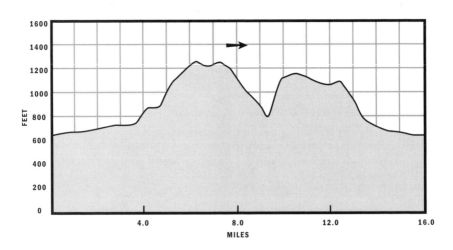

Levi or Paolo, that's another matter. Please disregard the previous words of caution.

From the intersection of Woodman Avenue and Ventura Boulevard, begin riding west. In this part of Sherman Oaks, Ventura Boulevard is lined with lots of proprietor-run shops and restaurants. It's a refreshing switch from the commercial developments and their strings of big-box retailers. There's plenty to look at, and you are very likely to notice a shop or restaurant you'll want to visit later in the day.

For most of the week, Ventura is a very busy street. This isn't a ride to do during rush hour. You'll have no trouble with traffic, though, if you tackle this on a weekend morning. That said, there's still a high probability that somebody in an overpowered German sedan will pass you at speeds better suited to interstellar travel. Stay to the right and you should be OK. Because Ventura is so heavily traveled, you'll notice that the road condition isn't the best; keep an eye out for large cracks in the pavement.

Your route climbs slightly as you ride west through Sherman Oaks toward Encino.

The change of communities will be easy to notice. Development turns suddenly large. Office buildings and strip malls replace the small shops and restaurants. After just more than 2 miles, you pass beneath I-405. The tunnel isn't long, but traffic changing lanes to the right to enter the 405 southbound won't be watching for you. Maintain a good lookout to your left and behind you as you pass beneath the freeway.

At the 3.6-mile mark, turn left onto Hayvenhurst Avenue. The very gentle false flat you have been warming up on becomes a more distinct climb at this point, though at 3.4 percent, the grade isn't bad. Don't make the mistake of going hard now just because the climb isn't steep; that's going to change later, and you want to save something for the coming challenge. A half-mile into the climb, Hayvenhurst turns 90 degrees to the right; be sure to follow it. Hayvenhurst immediately turns left again and resumes climbing.

You'll notice that, as you climb, the road gradually turns steeper. Eventually, you see a sign that says the road ahead dead-ends, and an arrow points left for Mulholland Drive. Turn left here onto Calneva Drive. The climb to Mulholland is a mere 0.6 miles, but it is the steepest climb of more than a half-mile in LA County. At an average gradient of 13.6 percent and with pitches that hit 18 percent, this ride might be the perfect tune-up for the Fargo Street challenge on page 128. If you are armed with a triple, make sure you downshift before you make the turn because once you are climbing the steep grade it is unlikely any derailleur will respond to shifter input.

Calneva Drive dead-ends at Mulholland. Turn left and take a breather as you freewheel; the road heads downhill on a gentle grade. In the next half-mile, you pass several churches. If you choose to ride on a Sunday, be mindful of the churchgoers as they come and go; there are likely to be a number of drivers on the road at the same time. After passing the last of the churches, the road turns down more dramatically before passing over the 405. Once you are past Rimerton Road, the asphalt turns skyward again. Drivers headed for the 405

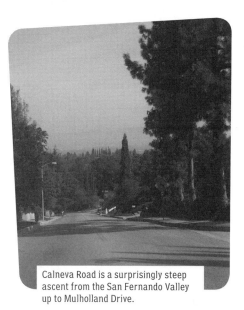

Calneva Road is a surprisingly steep ascent from the San Fernando Valley up to Mulholland Drive.

turn right on Rimerton; traffic will drop off as you begin your ascent. This hill is only 0.4 miles but does its damage in two short, steep kicks.

Just as the road levels off once again, turn left onto Longbow Drive. You won't see the road until you are right at the turn; in your approach, it is shielded from view by a large earthen berm. The road switchbacks right and left before you turn left onto Scadlock Lane, a road situated precariously above the 405, which it parallels. The 1.25-mile descent doesn't wind much and averages 8 percent. It can be quite steep at times, so watch for traffic entering from driveways.

Scadlock dead-ends at Deerhorn Drive. Turn right, immediately left onto Woodcliff Road, and immediately right on Rayneta Drive, which begins climbing with surprising suddenness. Following a right-hand bend, Rayneta turns left, but the main road continues straight and the name changes to Cody Road. Continue straight on Cody. The real surprise of this climb is how much the skyscraper cliffs and overhanging homes serpentined up the road evoke parts of the French Riviera where the mountains run to the sea. With views like this, summertime triple-digit temperatures seem worth it.

On your way up Cody, you encounter half a dozen large speed bumps (each roughly 3 feet across); chances are you won't be speeding, and the slope of the bumps isn't so great as to disturb you much. The climb hits grades as steep as 15 percent at times. All this black-diamond stuff has the net effect of yielding some extraordinary views on occasion; watch for opportunities to your left.

Cody Road eventually dead-ends into Woodcliff Road. Dig in for this final, steep (14-percent) push to Mulholland Drive. Turn left and take a breather as you enjoy the brief downhill. The shoulder here is not of consis-

Views here are of homes that each benefited from the hand of an individual architect rather than the cookie-cutter stamp of a developer. The ride also boasts the steepest climb of more than a half-mile in LA County, Calneva Drive, which makes for an excellent challenge early in the ride.

tent width; at times it is as wide as 6 feet, but at other times it is less than two 2 wide. Stay to the right should someone decide to use Mulholland for bobsled practice.

At the light at Beverly Glen Drive, turn left. Turn right on Coy Drive almost immediately. Beverly Glen is a fairly busy road, and this will get you out of the traffic flow. The pavement on Cody isn't exactly the best, but the nearly nonexistent traffic makes it worthwhile. Following a tight right switchback, turn left on Camino de la Cumbre. As you make the left, be mindful of the water channel molded into the concrete to guide runoff through the intersection; hit the wrong way, this could send you to the deck abruptly. The road is steep here and continues that way for most of the descent.

Camino de la Cumbre is a tiny residential street carved from the hillside on the left and overlooks the canyon to the right. Views range between peaceful and wow.

At Valley Vista Boulevard, turn right. This road is residential but is used as a secondary route when Ventura Boulevard is backed up. Provided you are doing this ride on a weekend morning, traffic should be light. The road continues downhill for the most part, but the grade is much gentler. While the homes here are very nice, many of them are much more understated in their beauty than are those up in the hills. These evoke less of Monte Carlo than they do of *Leave It to Beaver*. Almost exactly 1.5 miles from your last turn (at 13.1 miles), Valley Vista curves left and meets Ventura Boulevard. Turn left here and pedal the final 0.8 miles back to the ride's start.

After the Ride
With so many neat shops and restaurants in the area, it would be a shame to get back in your car right away. This part of Sherman Oaks is refreshingly quaint. Have lunch, check out some of the shops, and maybe drive back up to Mulholland for a final view of the San Fernando Valley.

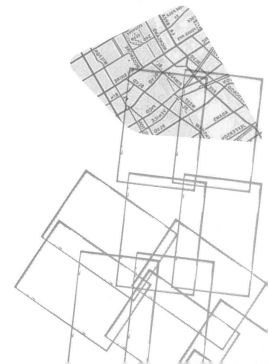

33 The Simi Ride

AT A GLANCE

Length: 57.5 miles
Configuration: Loop
Difficulty: Difficult
Climbing: 3,800 feet

Maximum gradient: 8%

Scenery: Suburbia, canyons, desert rock, and multicolored Lycra

Exposure: Extreme

Road traffic: Moderate

Road surface: Good

Riding time: 3.25 hours

Maps: Los Angeles County *Thomas Guide* pages 500, 499, 529, 588, 589, and 559 and Ventura County *Thomas Guide* pages 498, 497, 527, 496, 526, 527, 556, 557, and 558

In Brief

The Simi Ride is arguably LA's most famous group ride. It serves primarily as an off-season training ride for racers. Along with the Montrose Ride and the Donut Ride, Simi is one of the three fastest rides in Los Angeles County. The loop takes in Simi Valley, Calabasas, and the far western edge of the San Fernando Valley. There are four versions of the Simi Ride, ranging from 55 to 75 miles.

Directions

Many riders who do the Simi Ride live in Los Angeles and so choose to start the ride from the San Fernando Valley rather than from Simi Valley because San Fernando is more convenient for them. From the interchange of CA 101 and I-405, drive north 6.5 miles on the 405, then take CA 118 west 8 miles and exit at Topanga Canyon Boulevard. Take Topanga Canyon 2 miles south to Lassen Street. There

is plenty of free street parking on both Topanga Canyon and Lassen.

Description

For avid roadies, the Simi Ride is a right of passage. It is best known as the training ride for the Mercury Cycling Team during its heyday. Started by the former Masters' National Champion Barry Wolfe in the early 1970s, it has drawn many of the sport's top riders over the years. Attendees have included Greg LeMond, Giro d'Italia winners Andy Hampsten and Pavel Tonkov, Floyd Landis, Chris Horner, Henk Vogels, the local legend Thurlow Rogers, and seemingly every aspiring Category II racer in Southern California.

This ride does deviate from the selection criteria for group rides in a few ways. First, it does not occur year-round. During the summer months, much of the area gets too hot for all but the earliest rides. Second, the route does change over the course of the

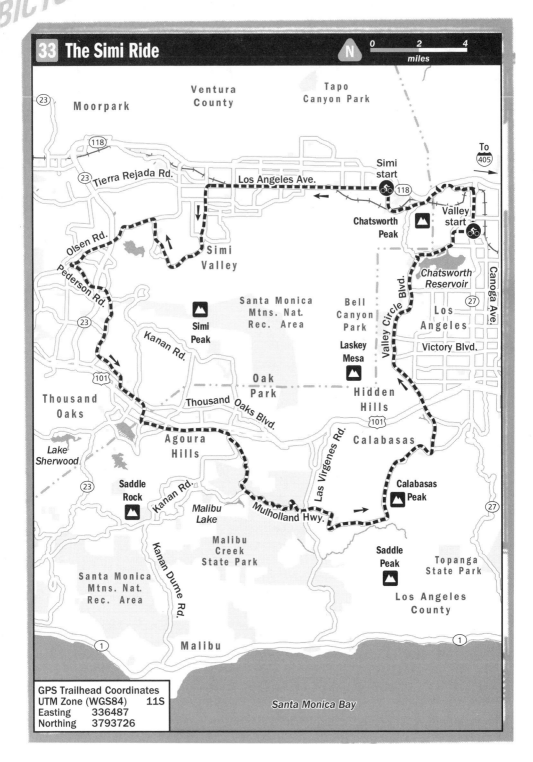

33 **The Simi Ride**

N

0   2   4
miles

Moorpark

Ventura
County

Tapo
Canyon Park

To
405

23

118

23   Tierra Rejada Rd.

Los Angeles Ave.

Simi
start

118

Simi
Valley

Olsen Rd.

Pederson Rd.

Chatsworth
Peak

Valley
start

Chatsworth
Reservoir

Canoga Ave.

Simi
Peak

Santa Monica
Mtns. Nat.
Rec. Area

Bell
Canyon
Park

Valley Circle Blvd.

Los
Angeles

27

23

Kanan Rd.

Laskey
Mesa

Victory Blvd.

101

Oak
Park

Thousand Oaks Blvd.

Hidden
Hills

Thousand
Oaks

Agoura
Hills

101

Las Virgenes Rd.

Calabasas

Lake
Sherwood

23

Kanan Rd.

Saddle
Rock

Malibu
Lake

Mulholland Hwy.

Calabasas
Peak

27

Kanan Dume Rd.

Malibu
Creek
State Park

Saddle
Peak

Topanga
State Park

Santa Monica
Mtns. Nat.
Rec. Area

Los Angeles
County

1

1

Malibu

Santa Monica Bay

GPS Trailhead Coordinates
UTM Zone (WGS84)   11S
Easting   336487
Northing   3793726

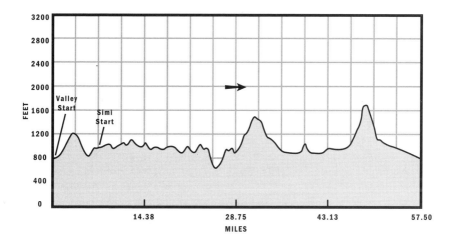

season. Third, more than half of its mileage is outside LA County. Despite those strikes against it, this guide would have been incomplete without this ride.

The course has changed a bit since its inception because roads have changed or become impractical, but it remains as faithful as possible to its original layout. Through the course of the off-season, when this ride sees its greatest attendance, the peloton can number anywhere from 80 riders to upward of 200. Despite the ride's large size, it is generally considered safe; if anyone gets out of line, more-experienced riders will set him or her straight.

Many riders who participate in this ride meet in the San Fernando Valley at Lassen and Topanga as it is more convenient (than Simi Valley) to most of Los Angeles. Riders departing Lassen and Topanga leave as early as 7:45 a.m., but most wait until 8 to begin the 15-minute spin to the ride's official start on Los Angeles Avenue. Ride 1.3 miles north on Topanga Canyon Boulevard and turn left on Old Santa Susana Pass

Road. This road runs flat initially but, following a left bend, begins climbing the rest of its half-mile ascent to Santa Susana Pass Road. Turn left there and continue climbing. The next 2 miles rise 664 feet to Santa Susana Pass at a 5-percent grade.

The descent is easy. Aside from a few cracks in the road surface, there are no surprises; the gentle curves of the road don't require braking even once. Santa Susana Pass becomes Kuehner Drive and eventually Los Angeles Avenue. Los Angeles straightens to run north, and at the 6.2-mile mark, you will see a sign indicating Los Angeles Avenue's left turn; move into the left lane and make the turn to continue on Los Angeles. Immediately after the turn, pull off at Dowel Drive, at your right. This is the Simi Ride's official meeting point. In the next 15 minutes or so, riders will arrive from every direction.

For the first 6.8 miles, you descend. If by any chance you aren't warmed up, this will give you adequate opportunity to do so. The gentle downhill allows the group to spin easily and lets members chat while maintaining a 20-mph pace. Los Angeles is seven lanes wide, but the group generally refrains from entering a second lane; the tactic is soundly discouraged and has gotten the entire ride pulled over—and ticketed—before. At First Street, the group turns left, finishing the runout of the downhill and rolling into the first real hill with the fully composed group. The climb up First is 2.5 miles but won't break legs with its 3-percent grade; it's essentially a false flat with a dash of spice.

Cresting the top, the descent begins immediately; a half-mile later, turn right on Wood Ranch Parkway. There is one brief rise interrupting the 2-mile descent. For better or worse, the next hill begins immediately. Downshift a few cogs, but don't leave the big ring. Turn left on Country Club Drive and continue to climb to the light at Madera Road. The group stops until it is appropriate to turn.

The next 3 miles are anything but flat, though you won't experience any significant hills either. Madera becomes East Olsen Road as the group heads for the next turn at Pederson Road. In the group, you aren't likely to see much of the sights, which at this point mostly consist of housing developments and nearby hills. The good news is that inside the bubble of the peloton, the constant rolling terrain will feel a lot flatter because you won't

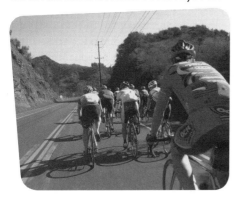

have to face the wind alone. At this point, you have left Simi Valley and are now riding through Thousand Oaks.

The group turns left at Erbes Road. As to the terrain, let's just say they didn't bulldoze quite everything. There's not a flat spot on this 3.5 miles of Erbes. Turn right on Duesenberb Drive, then turn left on Thousand Oaks Boulevard less than a half-mile later. Thousand Oaks is a large boulevard but, again, the group works to occupy only the right lane. A mile later, turn right on Lakeview Canyon Road, which takes you south over US 101. You'll pass a golf course and turn left on Agoura Road to continue paralleling the golf course (at your left), but you'll likely never notice it. Over the next 3.4 miles, Agoura continues to parallel the 101 and will climb one small hill, level off, and then descend to the next turn. By now, 33 miles into the ride, a pattern should be emerging: The flats and descents are soft pedaled, whereas you ride the hills at a firm tempo.

Turn right on Cornell Road; this will take you from the sprawling suburbia of LA's bedroom communities and into the Santa Monica Mountains. Cornell leads you 2.5 miles to your big rendezvous of the day: the Mulholland Hills. The Simi Ride uses a short portion of Mulholland Highway, portrayed more fully in the Mulholland Highway Loop ride on page 2.

Turn left on Mulholland. You immediately encounter two tough hills that will begin the process of shedding slower riders. Be prepared to make some big efforts on these hills. The hills are each roughly 0.6 miles long. The road continues to undulate before plunging down a rollicking descent, losing nearly 500 feet of elevation in only 1.2 miles. Do not allow yourself to be gapped before entering this descent; if you are, you will find your nose in the wind as you watch the group roll away at 40 mph. Despite the twists of the road on this descent, the broad sweeping turns enable you to stay on the gas full time. Be ready to use that 12.

Mulholland kicks up slightly a few hundred meters before reaching the intersection with Las Virgenes. The light here is the saving grace for many riders, allowing them to rejoin the group. The reunion is usually short-lived, though. After crossing Las Virgenes, you encounter what is for all practical purposes a 6-mile climb. The climb is broken by several brief downhills, but the speed of the group is such that if you get dropped, there is no chance of rejoining before the top of the climb. The good news: the group stops at the top. You gain the 880 feet of elevation on a measly 3-percent grade, but that won't matter. Climb with everything you've got to stay with the group.

Mulholland bends left and rises slightly as you approach the left turn on Dry Canyon Cold Creek Road. The Simi Ride calls this 2-mile climb Seven Minute Hill. Don't worry, many riders send up the white flag the moment they turn onto the climb, and simply ride at their own pace and watch the group ride off around a corner.

At the top, have a bite to eat and take a few pulls from your bottle. With 45 miles of the ride complete, you are likely in need of calories and don't want to risk bonking during the final 12. If you need water, there is a spigot behind the guardhouse (for the gated community) at the top of the climb. After a few minutes' rest, one of the ride's elders calls everyone to roll out.

Descend 2 miles to Old Topanga Canyon Boulevard and turn left. Old Topanga bends left and becomes Valmar Road. Just a hundred meters farther, turn left on Mulholland Drive and recross the 101. You are back in the San Fernando Valley now. Mulholland changes to Valley Circle Boulevard and continues northwest. The next 3.5 miles

on Valley Circle are likely the flattest of the entire ride. Here, at the very western edge of the San Fernando Valley, traffic is lighter and the wide right lane gives the group the room it needs to head for the final climb of the ride. The hill up Valley Circle is only a half-mile, but this late in the game and ascending at a 6-percent grade, it's a leg-breaker. Hang on, and over the top you'll be able to roll into a descent for recovery.

After 0.6 miles of descending, the road flattens once again for nearly 2 miles of easy cruising. Valley Circle will turn right and become Lake Manor Drive. Be sure to stay to the right because another road, Box Canyon, will be merging from your left. Box Canyon is a great climb you might want to try on your own. After 0.6 miles, Lake Manor becomes Valley Circle once again. Don't worry; that doesn't last. Valley Circle kinks right to become Plummer, and you turn left on Baden Avenue. Half a mile later, turn right at Lassen. Those riders returning to Simi Valley will continue straight, but a number of riders will turn right with you and spin easy for the final 0.75 miles back to Topanga Canyon. It's not much of a cooldown, but no one ever complains.

After the Ride

Once you have finished the Simi Ride, it is unlikely you will be concerned with much other than food. Most of Topanga Canyon is lined with restaurants. Many riders will get a bite at one of the places at the intersection of Topanga Canyon and Lassen. It's a great opportunity to pick up strategies for the ride and to get to know your new friends.

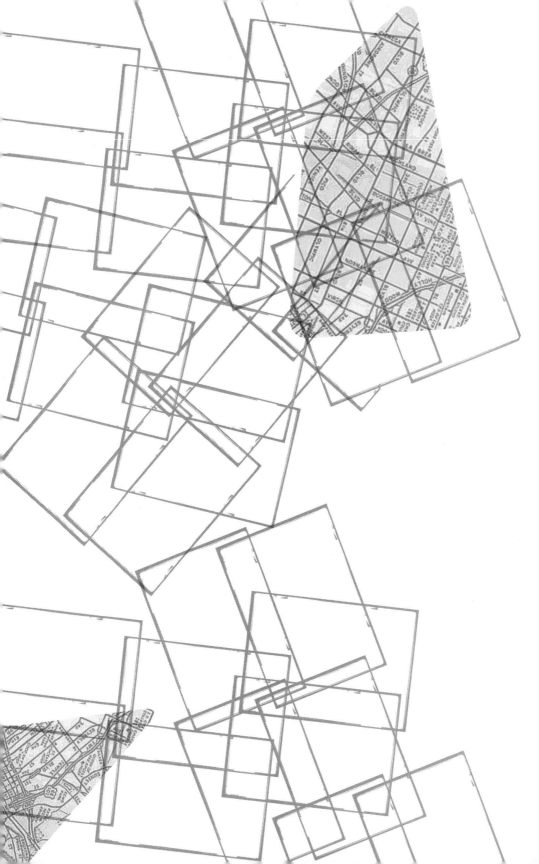

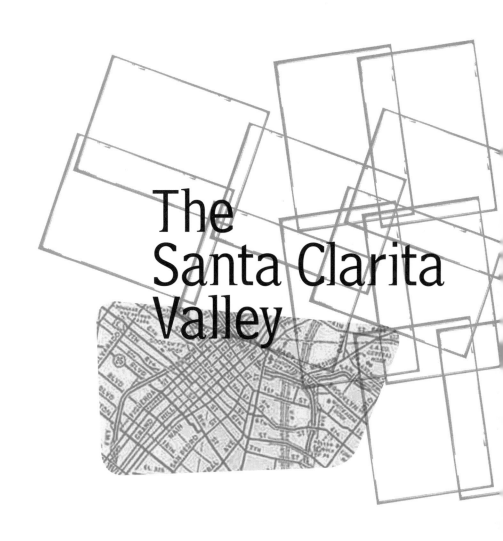

The
Santa Clarita
Valley

34 Bouquet Canyon Loop

AT A GLANCE

Length: 45 miles
Configuration: Loop
Difficulty: Difficult
Climbing: 3,700 feet

Maximum gradient: 10%
Scenery: Desert foliage, the Angeles National Forest, mountains
Exposure: Extreme
Road traffic: Light, except for the first few miles of Bouquet Canyon
Road surface: Good
Riding time: 3 hours
Maps: Los Angeles County *Thomas Guide*
pages 4550, 4551, 4461, 4281, 4283, 4193, 4192, F, 4279, and 4460

In Brief

This ride goes into the mountainous desert region north of the Santa Clarita Valley, a surprisingly remote area, given its overall proximity to Los Angeles. The northern end of the course takes riders by Bouquet Reservoir, up the surprisingly difficult Spunky Canyon, and through the small enclave of Green Valley. The trip returns via San Francisquito Canyon.

Description

From the parking structure, take Circle Drive north to the intersection of Auto Center Drive and Magic Mountain Parkway. At the right of the intersection, there is an entrance to the bike path and a ramp to a bridge that spans Magic Mountain Parkway. Take the bike path north, over Creekside Boulevard, until it intersects the main section of bike path.

Directions

From the intersection of I-5 and I-405 in the San Fernando Valley, drive north 10.6 miles on I-5 and exit at Valencia Boulevard. Take Valencia 1 mile to McBean Parkway. Turn left on McBean, and then turn right at the first light, at Town Center Drive. At the stop sign, turn left and head into the parking structure.

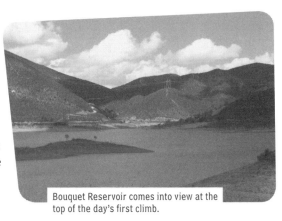

Bouquet Reservoir comes into view at the top of the day's first climb.

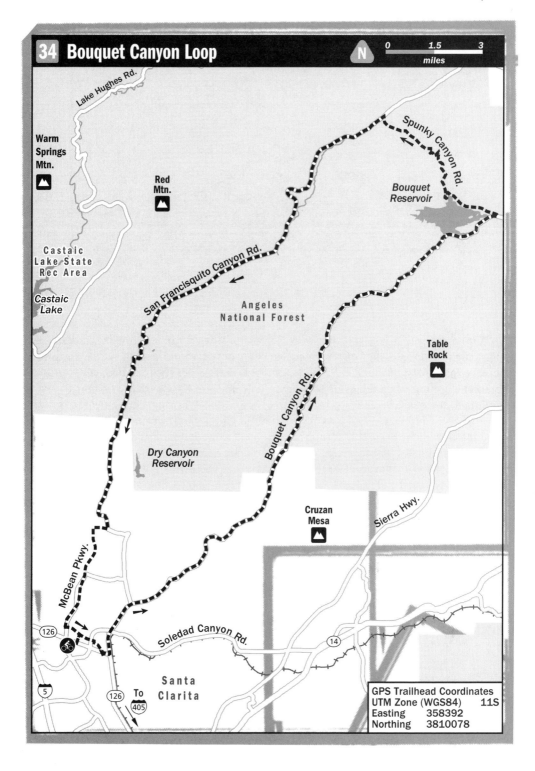

34 Bouquet Canyon Loop

N

0   1.5   3
miles

Lake Hughes Rd.

Spunky Canyon Rd.

Warm
Springs
Mtn.

Red
Mtn.

Bouquet
Reservoir

Castaic
Lake State
Rec Area

San Francisquito Canyon Rd.

Angeles
National Forest

Castaic
Lake

Table
Rock

Bouquet Canyon Rd.

Dry Canyon
Reservoir

McBean Pkwy.

Cruzan
Mesa

Sierra Hwy.

126

Soledad Canyon Rd.

14

Santa
Clarita

5

126   To
405

GPS Trailhead Coordinates
UTM Zone (WGS84)   11S
Easting   358392
Northing   3810078

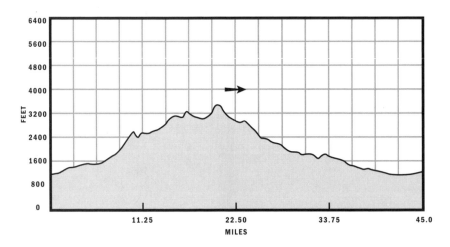

Turn right onto the bike path. Ride 1 mile on the path, passing under Valencia Boulevard and Magic Mountain Parkway. As you come up from the underpass of Magic Mountain, there will be chain-link fence to your right separating a gravel parking area from the bike path. Make a U-turn around the fence, and take the driveway to Magic Mountain Parkway. Turn right onto Magic Mountain. A little more than 100 yards later, Magic Mountain intersects Bouquet Canyon Road. Two lanes of traffic turn left onto Bouquet Canyon; move into the right of the two turn lanes. As you turn, you will be able to move easily to the wide shoulder and away from the traffic. Bouquet Canyon is busy thoroughfare. Even though you won't be on major streets in Valencia for very long, this ride is best enjoyed either very early in the day (any day of the week) or after 10 a.m. on weekdays.

Continue riding northeast on Bouquet Canyon. Traffic will ease just before you pass Seco Canyon Road 0.7 miles after your turn onto Bouquet Canyon; a bike lane begins there. After 8.5 miles, you'll pass Vazquez Canyon Road and should notice considerably less traffic. The road here edges gradually upward; the opening 17.5 miles of this ride average, amazingly, a 2-percent grade. The climb won't get noticeably more difficult until you pass the US Forest Service office at 10.5 miles.

The scenery here is surprisingly lush for the area. Tree cover is especially rare in this region, and on a hot day it can make the climb much more bearable. The grade will continue to increase until the final mile of the climb, where it reaches 8.5 percent. If you began the climb with too much gusto, this final mile will serve as cruel punctuation to a long effort.

At roughly 18.8 miles, the climb will end. Pull off the road to the left. There is a small gravel parking area where you can recover from your effort. From this vantage, you can look down on Bouquet Reservoir and across it to the next challenge of your ride: Spunky Canyon. Take the opportunity to have a bite to eat while you are looking around.

After you roll away from the parking area, the road will rise slightly before relaxing into a short descent. Spunky Canyon Road will appear at your left just as you clear the edge of the reservoir. Turn left and enjoy the flat for the next 1.75 miles. The road will switchback around the northern shore of the reservoir, and as you enter the next switchback the asphalt will kick up severely.

The climb up Spunky Canyon rises roughly 420 feet in a single mile for an average gradient of 8 percent. The incline pitches upward mercilessly—until you reach the top, there is no recovery. From here, you view Jupiter Mountain to the west, rising to 4,300 feet; the Angeles National Forest is visible in all directions.

While this route can be completed in either direction, one of the biggest reasons for climbing the south side of Spunky Canyon is that descending the north side isn't nearly as difficult as descending the south side. The north side eases you into Green Valley at just slightly more than 4

percent, making the twists and turns of the descent much more enjoyable.

Once the road flattens in Green Valley, you will notice a small convenience store to your left. This is your only opportunity to get water or an energy drink during the ride. And because temperatures can easily hit triple digits during the summer, staying hydrated takes some work.

From the store, ride two blocks to the intersection of Spunky Canyon and San Francisquito Canyon Road. Turn left on San Francisquito Canyon and begin to descend. The early portion of this descent turns little but is rather steep. Speeds upward of 45 mph are easy to achieve on the 2.2-mile descent if you let the bike run. Should you opt out of brake use, move toward the center of the lane; deer, small mammals, and reptiles can wander into the road, and, should that happen, you want as much room to work with as possible.

Immediately after you reach the bottom, the road kicks back up for a short (0.4-mile) rise. You pass beneath a set of large pipes

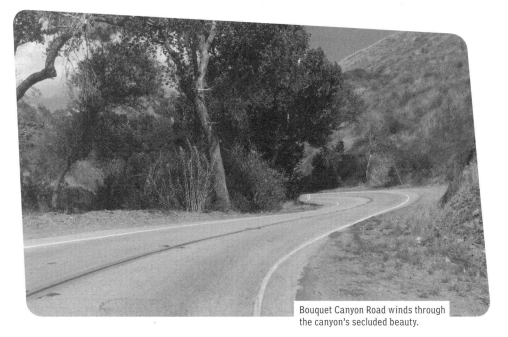

Bouquet Canyon Road winds through the canyon's secluded beauty.

for the California Aqueduct, which brings water from Central California into the Los Angeles basin.

After passing the pipes, the descent resumes. For the next 13.5 miles, the road descends more than 1,300 feet. Although this works out to a measly 2-percent grade, understand that the gradient on the 2 miles following the pipes is much closer to 5 or 6 percent. Turns are few, and, because the road was resurfaced relatively recently, if you take the turns properly, you won't need to touch the brakes.

Lower down the canyon, the road runs almost imperceptibly downhill for the most part, giving your pace a one-to-two cog advantage (that is, the downhill will give the rider enough advantage to be able to upshift one to two cogs depending on the rider's strength). There are a few short rises, but the biggest determinant of your pace will be the wind. On many days, a wind can begin running up the canyon around noon and utterly eliminate the downhill advantage.

You pass very near the site of the old San Francisquito Dam, which burst back in the 1920s. Mulholland's great engineering mistake washed billions of gallons of water down this canyon and into the Santa Clara River, ultimately destroying everything in its path—including the town of Piru—on its way to the Pacific.

At the bottom of the canyon, the point at which all the water from the dam turned right, the road begins to climb back up. Following a 90-degree bend to the left, the grade increases to 6 percent; soon after, you'll encounter a bend back to the right for the last of the climb up to Copper Hill Drive.

Turn right on Copper Hill and take it three blocks to McBean Parkway. You can either turn left onto McBean or swing wide and ride up onto the bike path. Although it seems more like a glorified sidewalk than a bona fide bike path, it does help you avoid a lot of traffic. Take McBean (or the bike path) 2.9 miles, past Decoro Drive and Newhall Ranch Road. Immediately after you cross the bridge over the Santa Clara River, turn right for the entrance to rejoin the bike path. Pass through the opening in the fence and make the U-turn to take you back under McBean. Ride the final 0.1 mile to the right turn that will take you back to the mall.

Take a moment to slow down when you reach the second bridge and look out over Magic Mountain Parkway. It's an unusual view. Take it easy going down the ramp back to the parking lot; there is a bus stop at the bottom of the ramp, and there are usually people present.

After the Ride

There is plenty to keep you busy following your ride, whether you're looking for food, shopping, or recreation. The Valencia Town Center has a large shopping mall, numerous shops and restaurants, and a movie theater.

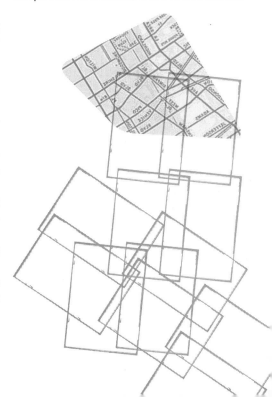

35 Lake Hughes Loop

AT A GLANCE

Length: 62 miles
Configuration: Loop
Difficulty: Difficult
Climbing: 4,300 feet

Maximum gradient: 12%

Scenery: Arid forest, desert

Exposure: Extreme

Road traffic: Mostly light

Road surface: Good

Riding time: 4.5 hours

Maps: Los Angeles County *Thomas Guide*
pages 4550, 4460, 4459, 4369, 4279, F, 4101, 4102, 4192, 4281, 4279, and 4460

In Brief

Lake Hughes sits in the high desert north of the Santa Clarita Valley and west of Palmdale. It is one the most sparsely populated regions of Los Angeles County. The ride begins with a flat spin from Valencia to Castaic Lake, whereupon the climbing starts. On the way out to Lake Hughes, the route climbs most of the way. The ride back descends through San Francisquito Canyon to its return in Valencia.

Directions

From the intersection of I-5 and I-405 in the San Fernando Valley, drive north 10.6 miles on I-5 and exit at Valencia Boulevard. Take Valencia 1 mile to McBean Parkway. Turn left on McBean and then turn right at the first light; the street is called Mall Entrance. At the stop sign, turn left and head into the parking structure.

Description

From the parking structure, take Circle Drive north to the intersection of Auto Center Drive and Magic Mountain Parkway. At the right of the intersection, there is an entrance to the bike path and a ramp to a bridge that spans Magic Mountain. Take the bike path north, over Creekside Boulevard, until it intersects the main section of bike path. The opening of this ride is very flat and gives you ample opportunity to warm up your legs before tackling your first big challenge.

Turn left onto the bike path and ride a half-mile west. Pass under McBean Parkway and, at the top of the rise, make a U-turn around the chain-link fence. You will bear right through a gate in the fence and immediately turn left to head north on the path. Here the path seems more like a sidewalk than a bike path, but given the six lanes of traffic on McBean, the path is preferable to the checkered-flag rush of SUVs. After less than 100 yards, turn left and follow the path behind a home

BICYCLING

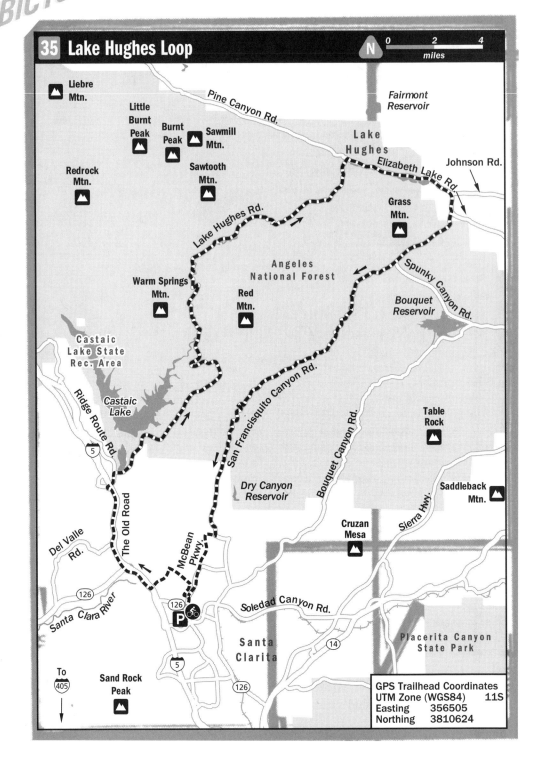

35 Lake Hughes Loop

N

0   2   4
miles

Liebre Mtn.

Little Burnt Peak

Burnt Peak

Sawmill Mtn.

Sawtooth Mtn.

Redrock Mtn.

Pine Canyon Rd.

Fairmont Reservoir

Lake Hughes

Elizabeth Lake Rd.

Johnson Rd.

Grass Mtn.

Lake Hughes Rd.

Angeles National Forest

Warm Springs Mtn.

Red Mtn.

Spunky Canyon Rd.

Bouquet Reservoir

Castaic Lake State Rec. Area

Castaic Lake

Ridge Route Rd.

5

San Francisquito Canyon Rd.

Table Rock

Bouquet Canyon Rd.

Dry Canyon Reservoir

Saddleback Mtn.

The Old Road

McBean Pkwy.

Del Valle Rd.

126

126

Santa Clara River

Cruzan Mesa

Sierra Hwy.

Soledad Canyon Rd.

5

Santa Clarita

14

Placerita Canyon State Park

To 405

Sand Rock Peak

126

GPS Trailhead Coordinates
UTM Zone (WGS84)   **11S**
Easting   356505
Northing   3810624

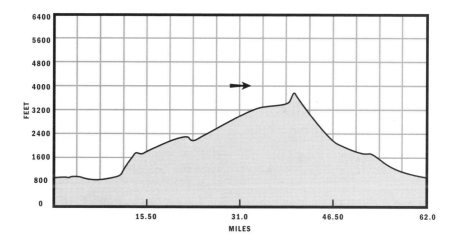

development. Here's where being on the bike path makes sense. The noise level drops, road debris is replaced by plants and mulch, and the worst traffic you'll find will consist of tricycles and baby carriages.

The path will pass under Bridgeport Lane then, a half-mile later, under Newhall Ranch Road. At the top of the rise, make a U-turn and take the path up to Newhall Ranch. Ride down the ramp and turn right onto that road. These four lanes are driven like almost all larger roads in the Santa Clarita Valley—as if the drivers' last names were Earnhart. Speeds upwards of 60 mph are common. The right lane is wide; just be sure to keep an eye out for trucks coloring outside the lines, so to speak. One mile from your turn onto Newhall Ranch, turn left on Rye Canyon Loop. Approximately 1.1 miles later, pass under I-5. Turn right on The Old Road and take it 5 miles to Ridge Route, then turn right. Just before the turn, the road rises slightly, and then Ridge Route runs downhill by a few restaurants and truck stops. This lasts a half mile. Turn right from Ridge Route onto Lake Hughes Road.

Immediately after the turn, cross the short bridge and downshift. The first big climb of the day begins here. The 2.5-mile climb ascends 910 feet for an average gradient of just less than 7 percent. It's really a rude awakening. That said, the views you gain of Lake Castaic are enough to distract you from the difficulty of your endeavor. The next 9 miles on this road undulate with the ridgeline. Views to the east and west take in classic rocky desert

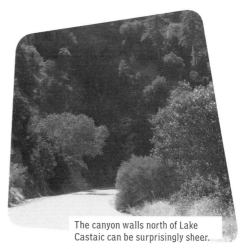

The canyon walls north of Lake Castaic can be surprisingly sheer.

The opening of this ride is very flat and gives you ample opportunity to warm up your legs before tackling your first big challenge.

landscapes with impossibly looming red sandstone formations dotting the otherwise sand-colored ground.

Following one quick dip with a banked, left curve at the bottom, downshift for the grind up to the top of the hill. To your left are your final and most impressive views of Lake Castaic. Over the top, quickly shift to your big ring and begin dumping your chain to your smallest cog. The descent here isn't too long—only 1.5 miles—but you have the opportunity to reach speeds in excess of 40 mph. Following a sweeping bend to the right, the road gives way to a short concrete bridge that marks the end of your free ride.

The next 10 miles of the ride are almost continuously uphill. While your name doesn't have to be Zabriskie to take this 3-percent grade in the big ring, it might help. It's easy to start out kicking through each rise and recovering on the short flats, but blowing up before the turn on Elizabeth Lake Road can make for a rather long day. Cool it here and save something for the climb up San Francisquito.

At Elizabeth Lake Road, turn right. A short distance after passing much of the town and Hughes Lake, you'll see this Lilliputian community's one store on your right. If you need more snacks or water, or something stronger, this is the place to get it. You won't have another opportunity

until you return to Valencia.

At the 38-mile mark, Elizabeth Lake Road forks. To your left is Johnson Road. Stay right on Elizabeth Lake. A very short downhill runout from the turn adds a little punch to your pedal stroke. Another 0.8 miles on, turn right on San Francisquito Canyon Road. This climb is short—only 1.2 miles—but it ascends nearly 600 feet for an average grade of 9 percent and tops out at 3,932 feet, the ride's highest elevation. This little suffer-fest is peppered with some steeps, including a section at 12 percent.

The good news is that the downhill gives you back all you earned. The first mile averages roughly 12 percent—definitely steep for a descent, but its saving grace is its lack of turns. Even on days when a wind blows north through the canyon, coasting speeds can easily exceed 45 mph. Although the first 2 miles of the descent have no turns whatsoever, there is a stop sign at Spunky Canyon Road. Given the downhill grade, brake early for this stop. Traffic is light up here, but there tends to be some traffic at this intersection—skidding past the sign might not turn out well.

San Francisquito Canyon is a rather deceptive road. In general, the road descends back to Valencia. However, in its 18-mile run back to town, the road kicks up by various degrees no fewer than eight times. These rises are short; only one, the sixth, is longer than a half-mile, and it has caused many riders to mutter, "You've got to be kidding." It may well be one of the least-downhill descents around. Turns are few, though there is one important one to be aware of. At the 50-mile mark, San Francisquito Canyon goes straight at the point of a previous bend. This you aren't likely to notice, but the sharp left turn 2 miles later comes up suddenly. Fortunately, there's a stop sign here serving to prevent drivers and cyclists alike from overcooking the turn over a bridge and winding up in the creek below. This is, roughly, the location where William Mulholland built the dam that famously failed.

The road continues to wind for the next 2 miles before resuming its essentially straight run to Valencia. At 57 miles, you will round a left bend to your last significant hill; it's a sweeping right that runs 0.4 miles to Copper Hill Drive and presents a great opportunity to kick one last time and see if your legs have anything left. Turn right and coast downhill. Past the light at Canterbury Court, move to the left lane to turn left on McBean Parkway. McBean has two left-turn lanes, so stay in the right of the two lanes and immediately swing into the rightmost of the three lanes on McBean.

Roll down McBean the 3 miles to your turn back onto the bike path. One reason to tackle this ride either very early or after rush hour is to help time your return so that, when you are on McBean, traffic is as light as possible. After passing through the light at Newhall Ranch Road, you will cross the bridge over the Santa Clara River. Immediately beyond it is a ramp that will allow you to turn right beyond and pass through the chain-link fence surrounding the path.

After entering the path, make the U-turn to pass under McBean. One mile later, turn right at the intersecting path. After crossing the bridge over Magic Mountain Parkway, the path turns right and heads downhill to the bus stop. Take it easy through here; there tend to be a lot of people. Bear left into the Town Center parking complex, and head back to your car. No matter what time of year you do the ride, you'll be grateful for the covered parking.

After the Ride

There is plenty to keep you busy following your ride, whether you're looking for food, shopping, or recreation. The Valencia Town Center has a large shopping mall, numerous shops and restaurants, and a movie theater.

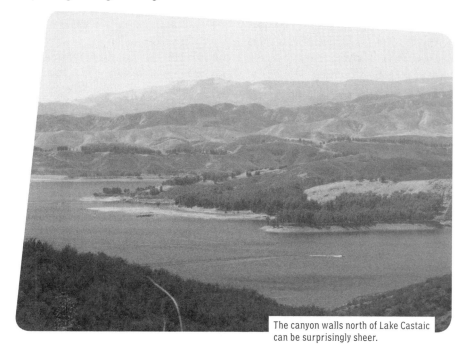

The canyon walls north of Lake Castaic can be surprisingly sheer.

36 Valencia Bike Paths

AT A GLANCE

Length: 9 miles
Configuration: Loop with spurs
Difficulty: Easy
Climbing: 200 feet

Maximum gradient: 8%

Scenery: Desert, dry riverbed, and ever-increasing commercial development

Exposure: Extreme

Road traffic: None

Road surface: Very good

Riding time: 1 hour

Maps: Los Angeles County *Thomas Guide*
pages 4550, 4551, and 4460

In Brief

The Santa Clarita Valley sits just north of the San Fernando Valley and has a climate noticeably more arid than much of the rest of Los Angeles. The community of Valencia planned a number of bike paths in the construction of the city. More than 17 miles of paths crisscross the area, and new sections are being added all the time.

Directions

From the intersection of I-5 and I-405 in the San Fernando Valley, drive north 10.6 miles on I-5 and exit at Valencia Boulevard. Take Valencia 1 mile to McBean Parkway. Turn left on McBean and then turn right at the first light, at Town Center Drive. At the stop sign, turn left and head into the parking structure.

Description

Valencia is a truly prefab community. Its development has been very carefully planned by a real estate–development corporation seeking to build a safe and (theoretically) affordable place for people to live and raise their families. At the center of the community is the "town center," a mall and shopping complex convenient to most residents. The arid, desert climate means temperatures can reach triple digits during the day for months on end. And although the old adage, "it's a dry heat," may work for you during the ride, you would be advised to park your car in the shade of a parking structure.

Views from many of the paths take in the (usually) dry bed of the Santa Clara River. Wildlife you may see in the area includes rabbits, several varieties of lizards, red-tailed hawks, turkey buzzards, and, occasionally, coyotes.

From the parking structure, take Circle Drive north to the intersection of Auto Center Drive and Magic Mountain Parkway. At the right of the intersection, there is an entrance to the bike path and

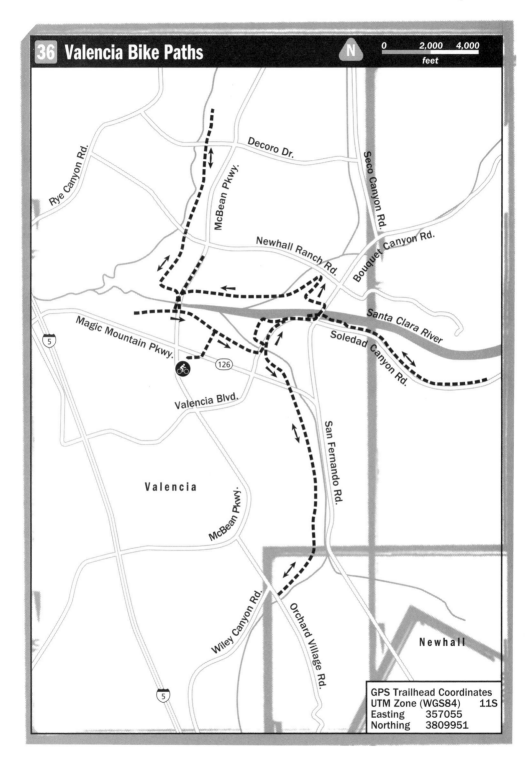

N

0   2,000   4,000
feet

Rye Canyon Rd.

Decoro Dr.

McBean Pkwy.

Seco Canyon Rd.

Newhall Ranch Rd.

Bouquet Canyon Rd.

Santa Clara River

Magic Mountain Pkwy.

5

126

Soledad Canyon Rd.

Valencia Blvd.

San Fernando Rd.

Valencia

McBean Pkwy.

Wiley Canyon Rd.

Orchard Village Rd.

Newhall

5

GPS Trailhead Coordinates
UTM Zone (WGS84)   11S
Easting   357055
Northing   3809951

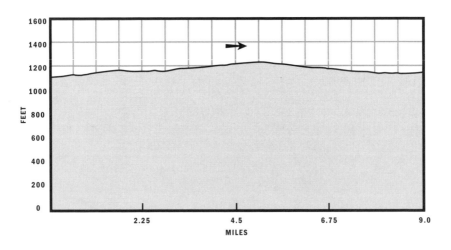

At each intersection, the bike path will pass either over or under the thoroughfare. The path passes beneath Valencia Boulevard and immediately turns right up a short hill. This is the steepest stretch you will encounter. At the top of the hill, the path bends right, and 0.4 miles later, it passes beneath Magic Mountain Parkway. The ramp isn't as steep as the last one, but without a sharp turn at the bottom, you can use your momentum heading back uphill so that it doesn't require much effort.

For the next 1.4 miles, an equestrian trail parallels the bike path on the side opposite the Santa Clara River. For the most part, there is undeveloped field for more than 100 yards beyond that, lending a much more secluded feeling to the ride.

Just 0.2 miles after the equestrian trail ends, there is an intersection. If you continue straight, the path terminates at Orchard Village Drive. If you turn left, the path crosses a bridge and ends at Newhall Avenue. Turn right and take the path around the short loop that will rejoin the bike path for your return trip. After crossing

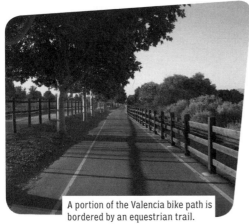
A portion of the Valencia bike path is bordered by an equestrian trail.

a ramp to a bridge that spans Magic Mountain. Take the bike path north, over Creekside Boulevard, until it intersects the main section of bike path.

Turn right and begin pedaling southwest along the path. This section of path parallels the Santa Clara River, which is usually drier than academia. Don't be surprised if you see a motorcycle or ATV cruising the sand. The foliage here is typical of the desert: piñon, desert sage, and other drought-resistant shrubs and bushes.

under Magic Mountain Parkway, the path curls left before the sharp right turn leading down the steep underpass of Valencia Boulevard. Use caution when the path turns left to pass below Valencia; the turn is slightly off-camber and not one you want to take too fast.

Just after you pass beneath the road is an opportunity to turn right and join a different path. The turn is sharp—almost 180 degrees—heading for Valencia Boulevard. Once the path reaches the street, you immediately encounter a left turn for another path. (While the path you are on continues, it parallels Valencia and isn't too scenic.) This second path is a half-mile detour around a commercial development and is much more scenic, what with the frightened bunnies darting across the path.

The path rejoins the section paralleling Valencia Boulevard; 0.2 miles later, things get a little weird, with the path ending at a gas station. To continue, ride along the sidewalk, watching for vehicles entering and leaving the parking lot. This aberration is mercifully brief—only 0.1 mile. Turn left at the corner and ride north; the path resumes just beyond the gas station. Your course parallels Bouquet Canyon Road as it crosses the Santa Clara River. Just another 100 yards or so up the path, it turns left and leaves Bouquet Canyon.

Almost immediately, the path turns right and heads north. To the left of the path is a large concrete culvert that feeds into the Santa Clara. At Newhall Ranch Road, the path turns parallel to the road momentarily before heading back down the other side of the culvert. At the Santa Clara, the path turns right and runs 1 mile to McBean Parkway. At this point, the course heads left, crosses the Santa Clara once again, and then turns left onto the bike path. Be careful as you pass through the chain-link fence.

From here it is 0.4 miles back to the intersection where you joined this path near the beginning of the ride. The intersection with the path back to the town center is unmarked, but you can tell it's the spot because the path passes between two auto dealerships. You'll notice a great many vehicles backed against the fence to the south as you near the turn. The final half-mile back to the parking structure begins with a very gentle uphill until you cross Magic Mountain Parkway and drop down from the bridge.

There are another 8 miles of bike path leading around the community of Valencia. In addition to that, Valencia has a network of paseos, paths smaller than a standard bike path but larger than sidewalks, where bicycling is permitted. They are well worth exploring and lead almost anywhere you might want to go in Valencia.

After the Ride

There is plenty to keep you busy following your ride, whether you're looking for food, shopping, or recreation. The Valencia Town Center has a large shopping mall, numerous shops and restaurants, and a movie theater.

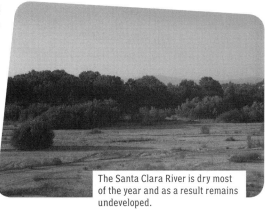

The Santa Clara River is dry most of the year and as a result remains undeveloped.

37 Vazquez Rocks Loop

AT A GLANCE

Length: 30 miles
Configuration: Loop
Difficulty: Moderate
Climbing: 1,500 feet

Maximum gradient: 7%

Scenery: Arid forest, desert

Exposure: Extreme

Road traffic: Mostly light

Road surface: Good

Riding time: 2.5 hours

Maps: Los Angeles County *Thomas Guide* pages 4373, 4463, 4464, 4465, and 4374

In Brief

This loop takes in the rocky, sandstone scenery of the desert in the eastern Santa Clarita Valley. The loop involves a fast, twisting descent followed by a surprisingly sustained climb that accounts for exactly half the ride. The scenery is both unusual and beautiful—and for fans of Coyote and the *Road Runner* cartoons, even comic at times.

Directions

From the intersection of I-5 and I-405 in the San Fernando Valley, drive north 3.5 miles, then take SR 14 north 14.5 miles. Exit at Agua Dulce Canyon Road, turn left at the bottom of the ramp, drive 1.6 miles, and turn right. You are still on Agua Dulce. At the stop sign 0.25 miles later, continue straight 0.4 miles, now on Escondido Canyon Road, then turn right into the entrance for Vazquez Rocks County Park.

Description

Your ride starts at Vazquez Rocks County Park. You know this place from countless Westerns, the odd *Star Trek* episode, and Reny Harlan's bloodbath *Starship Troopers*. When you step from your car, your first remark may well be that you've been here before. Vazquez Rocks' unusual appearance is due to the inclined layers of sandstone.

Turn left as you exit the driveway. You have a short, almost entirely flat roll to the turn on Agua Dulce Canyon Road. Turn left and begin descending. Agua Dulce Canyon is one of those rare roads that bends and turns with such gentle patience that a bicyclist need never apply the brakes. That's not idle talk: these roads were built for trucks— and perhaps their drivers' attitudes. For aggressive riders, it is possible to keep the power on for the entire descent without ever worrying that you might need to brake for a coming turn. These giant sweepers are the cyclist's equivalent of a Super G.

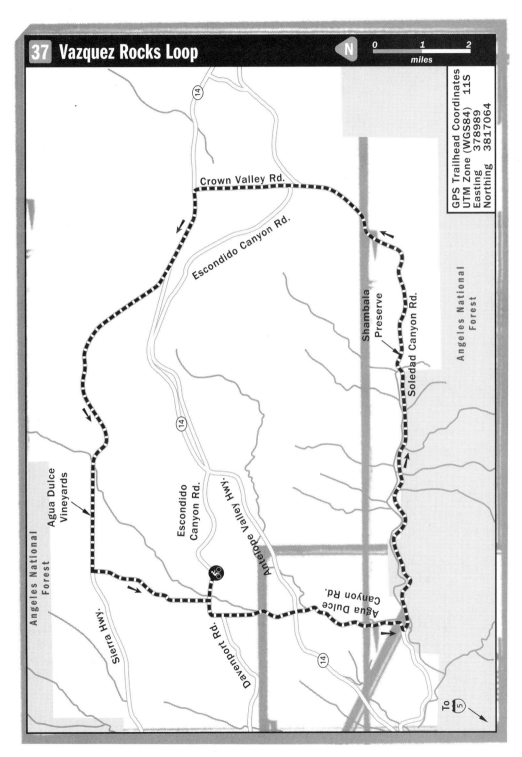

N

0   1   2
miles

GPS Trailhead Coordinates
UTM Zone (WGS84)   11S
Easting   378989
Northing   3817064

Crown Valley Rd.

Escondido Canyon Rd.

Shambala Preserve

Soledad Canyon Rd.

Angeles National Forest

Agua Dulce Vineyards

Escondido Canyon Rd.

Antelope Valley Hwy.

Agua Dulce Canyon Rd.

Angeles National Forest

Sierra Hwy.

Davenport Rd.

To 5

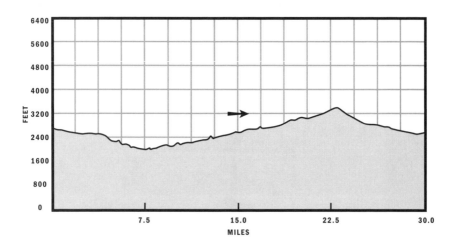

Now for the bad news: Every now and then, winds can kick up out of the south or east and funnel up this canyon, leaving a rider fighting for 30 mph on a road that would be more fun at 35. With an average gradient of less than 3 percent, this 4-mile descent can be defeated by a strong wind. An early departure is the best protection against the wind.

At 1.6 miles from the turn, you pass under SR 14 . Watch for traffic exiting the 14 both on your left and on your right. At the bottom of Agua Dulce, the road rises slightly before intersecting with Soledad Canyon Road. The left turn on Soledad Canyon is sharp—more than 90 degrees—and slightly off-camber. Because there is a

This loop takes in the rocky, sandstone scenery of the desert in the eastern Santa Clarita Valley.

stop sign at the intersection, none of this should be a problem.

Soledad Canyon begins what is essentially a 15-mile incline. At 1.8 percent in grade, this hardly constitutes a climb, but you will feel the 1,400-foot rise before it is over. The greater challenge to come will depend on the wind. With a headwind, you can be reduced to speeds that leave you thinking you must be climbing l'Alpe d'Huez.

If, as you ride, you hear the roaring of lions, don't be too surprised. Shambala Preserve, situated 10.2 miles into your loop, is Tippi Hedren's sanctuary for big cats. Shambala cares for a number of large cats, including lions, tigers, mountain lions, ligers (yes, they are real), and a cheetah, among others. While Ms. Hedren is best known for her role in Alfred Hitchcock's The Birds, it was her role in the 1981 movie Roar that first brought her in contact with the big cats. She has devoted her life to rescuing cats here in America ever since. Though the brush can obscure the view, it is possible to see a few of the compounds and the cats inside.

At 12.3 miles, you are faced with a choice.

Crown Valley Road forks off to the right. Soledad Canyon and Crown Valley will meet again in 2 miles. Go right on Crown Valley, and the route is flat and easy. Continue straight on Soledad Canyon and the asphalt spikes up over a short, steep hill. This stretch of road is regularly used for television commercials—mostly automotive stuff, but on one occasion a shoot involving cyclists. No matter which you choose, when you reach the second intersection of Soledad Canyon and Crown Valley (marked by the stop sign), ride north on Crown Valley. One block north is your first opportunity to fuel up if you need a drink or a snack; there is a small market to your right.

Crown Valley Road continues to climb gradually as your course takes you due north toward SR 14. While there is very little development on Soledad Canyon, Crown Valley is slightly more developed, with a number of side streets leading to homes. Traffic should still be pretty light, though.

After passing under CA 14, turn left on Sierra Highway, which will be the busiest of any of the roads you ride on. Don't worry: with its wide shoulder, traffic won't pass too close to you. Just when you think the climbing should be over, you get a bit of a surprise. There's still another 3.6 miles of climbing and 500 feet of elevation gain. With roughly 19 miles of the route covered, you finally get a break. Almost the entire rest of the ride is downhill, and what few hills you encounter are short and can be powered over in the big ring.

At 23.2 miles, you will come upon an unlikely sight: a grape vineyard. Agua Dulce Vineyards is one of Los Angeles County's only estate wineries, meaning that the winery grows grapes and ferments the juice into wine on site. While not every wine bearing Agua Dulce's label is local, with its 92 acres of vineyard, most of its offerings are. Seeing a vineyard in this desert is a truly unusual sight.

Turn left at Agua Dulce Canyon Road. The downhill run continues for the final 7 miles back to Vazquez Rocks. You'll pass through the enclave of Agua Dulce, where there is a market, an antique store, and a few restaurants.

After one final rise, you will reach the intersection at Escondido Canyon Road. Turn left for the final 0.4-mile ride back to Vazquez Rocks.

After the Ride
Following your ride, you have a number of fun options. By all means, take in a hike at Vazquez Rocks. Lunch can be found in Agua Dulce. Following lunch, you might consider a visit to Agua Dulce Vineyards. If you think you might like to check out the big cats at Shambala, be aware that tickets for the tours must be purchased in advance. You will need to plan your visit a few weeks ahead of time; they always sell out. It's a surprising number of options, given the remote location.

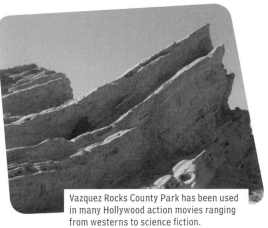

Vazquez Rocks County Park has been used in many Hollywood action movies ranging from westerns to science fiction.

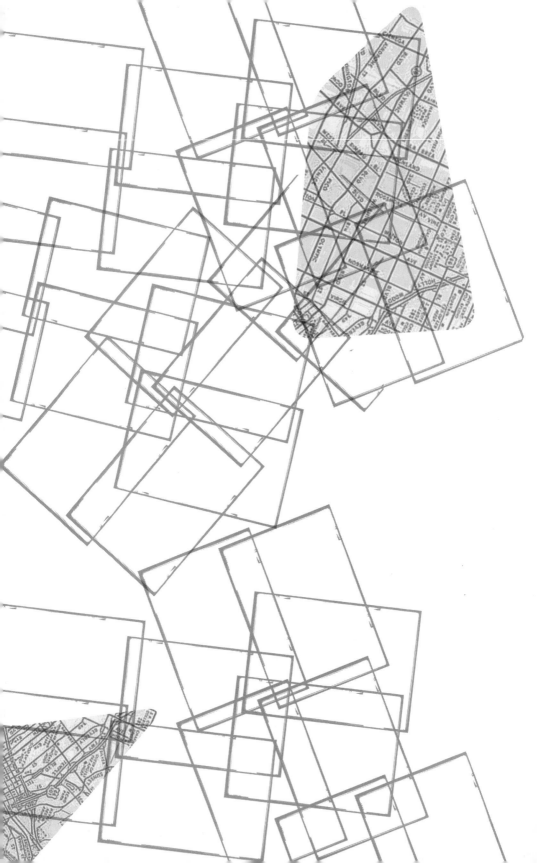

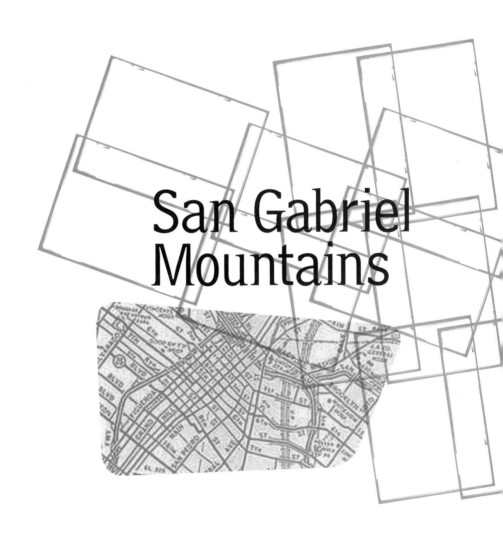

San Gabriel Mountains

38 Little Tujunga Loop

AT A GLANCE

Length: 51 miles
Configuration: Loop
Difficulty: Difficult
Climbing: 4,700 feet

Maximum gradient: 11%

Scenery: San Gabriel Mountains

Exposure: Severe

Road traffic: Light to fairly heavy

Road surface: Good to excellent

Riding time: 4 hours

Maps: Los Angeles County *Thomas Guide* pages 4550, 4640, 4641, 481, 482, 502, 4643, and 4642

In Brief

The Little Tujunga Loop takes you through the very western end of the San Gabriel Mountains. While some of the ride passes through an industrial area at the northern end of the San Fernando Valley, Little Tujunga Canyon Road offers riders two challenging climbs with stunning views of the neighboring peaks and arguably one of the most impressive views of the San Fernando Valley around.

Directions

From the intersection of I-5 and I-405 in the San Fernando Valley, drive north 10.6 miles on I-5, exiting at Valencia Boulevard. Take Valencia 1 mile to McBean Parkway, then turn left on McBean and then right at the first light; the street is called Mall Entrance. At the stop sign, turn left and head into the parking structure.

Description

Because it takes in a long stretch of road in a rather industrial area, this ride (like many others in this guide) is best done on weekend mornings. The industries will be closed and most of the nearby residents won't have risen yet. Traffic should be light for all but the final 2 miles of your ride. There is another reason to do this ride early: the Santa Clarita Valley heats up terribly during the day for a big chunk of the year. Consequently, this ride is most pleasant in spring and fall.

From the parking structure, take Circle Drive north to the intersection of Auto Center Drive and Magic Mountain Parkway. At the right of the intersection, there is an entrance to the bike path and a ramp to a bridge that spans Magic Mountain Parkway. Take the bike path north, over Creekside Boulevard, until it intersects the main section of bike path.

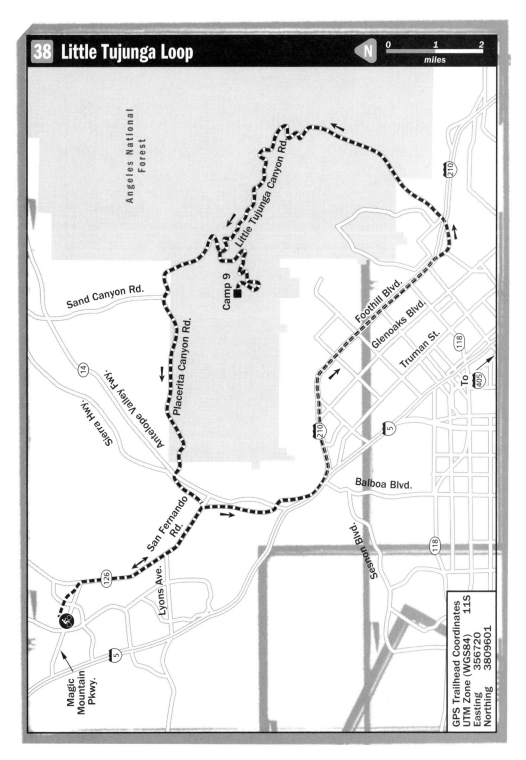

N

0   1   2
miles

Angeles National Forest

Little Tujunga Canyon Rd.

210

Sand Canyon Rd.

Camp 9

Foothill Blvd.

Glenoaks Blvd.

Placerita Canyon Rd.

Truman St.

118

To 405

14

Sierra Hwy.

Antelope Valley Fwy.

210

5

Balboa Blvd.

San Fernando Rd.

Sesnon Blvd.

118

126

Lyons Ave.

Magic Mountain Pkwy.

5

GPS Trailhead Coordinates
UTM Zone (WGS84)   11S
Easting   356720
Northing   3809601

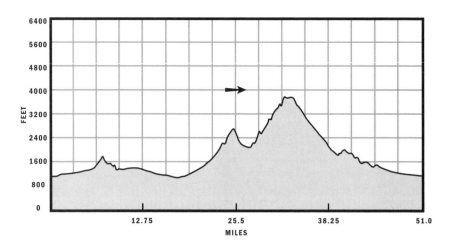

Turn right onto the bike path. Ride 1 mile on the path, passing under Valencia Boulevard and Magic Mountain Parkway. As you come up from the underpass of Magic Mountain, there will be chain-link fence to your right separating a gravel parking area from the bike path. Make a U-turn around the fence and take the driveway to Magic Mountain Parkway. Turn right onto Magic Mountain. A little more than 100 yards later, Magic Mountain intersects San Fernando Road. Turn right and begin riding southeast. San Fernando is a very, very slight false flat for the next 4 miles. It's a good warm-up, provided the wind isn't blowing in from the desert.

San Fernando is the major thoroughfare through the communities of Saugus and Newhall. These communities are closely associated with the Westerns of the 1950s; most of them were filmed in the area. On your right, just after your turn, the 100-year-old Saugus Café features photos of Roy Rogers and Gene Autry—one-time customers.

The shoulder is wide on San Fernando, so even if the SUVs pass you at freeway speeds, you shouldn't have serious fears for your safety. As you reach Newhall, the road will become narrower and the traffic a little heavier and slower. San Fernando will cut left slightly at the intersection with Newhall Road. Bear left and continue by William S. Hart Regional Park. You will encounter some railroad tracks as you pass the park; they cross the road at a less-than-90-degree angle; be careful as you cross them.

A mile past the railroad tracks, turn right onto Sierra Highway. With roughly 5.5 miles of the ride covered, your legs should be ready for the first hill of the day. Sierra also sports a wide shoulder, and, because it parallels CA 14, it is lightly traveled. The 1.5-mile climb tops out at roughly 1,800 feet as you cross San Fernando Pass.

Descend nearly a mile to Foothill Boulevard. This turn is easy to miss. Foothill intersects San Fernando from the left, emerging from beside CA 14. If you pass under CA 14, you have overshot the turn. The riding here isn't sexy, but passing this way allows you to get the biggest, busiest road out of the way early on. The next 9.5 miles are at least largely downhill, so the section passes quickly.

As you ride on Foothill, the San Gabriels loom just above you; the road parallels the mountains. When Foothill reaches Hansen Dam, it veers left. Pedal under I-210 and immediately turn left on Osborne Street.

Just off of Osborne, there is a convenience store on Lexicon Avenue. Should you want to get additional water, a sports drink, or a snack, get it here. This is your last chance for more than an hour.

The climb up Little Tujunga is a great challenge. The ascent begins mildly enough, and as you climb it will gradually get a bit steeper, but never terribly steep. The 7.3-mile ascent climbs more than 1,600 vertical feet at just more than a 4-percent average gradient. It doesn't turn and switchback as much as some climbs; focus on the road ahead and let the changes in view come to you.

At the 24.5-mile mark, just a third of a mile from the top of the climb, is an overlook. Stop for a moment; the vista of the surrounding peaks is remarkable, and your view takes in the road you have just climbed—it'll give you a great sense of accomplishment.

After you look around, spin the final piece of the climb and then shift into the big ring for the 2.25-mile descent of nearly 700 vertical feet. It's not a long drop, but the change feels good. The bottom is marked by a bridge across Pacoima Creek. Your rest is short-lived. Shift back into the small ring and get ready for the long climb of the day.

The climb up to Bear Divide and on to Camp 9 is 5.5 miles, ascends 1,750 feet, and averages a 6-percent grade. You encounter the nastiest, steepest stuff down low. After the left turn on Santa Clara Road (at 29 miles), the grade eases noticeably. Most riders can shift up a cog or two here. While it is possible to go straight and cut the ride short, doing so would be a huge mistake; the climb up Santa Clara to Camp 9 is too cool to miss.

Santa Clara is a road to nowhere—it goes to a fire station—so the road isn't used much. This explains why it, unlike almost every other road in this guide, is made from chip and seal. Simply put, it's a fancy gravel road. It's not as smooth as some roads, but it is serviceable.

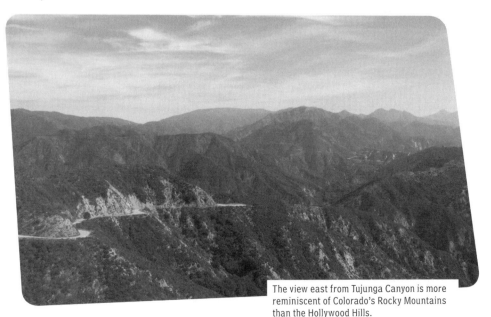

The view east from Tujunga Canyon is more reminiscent of Colorado's Rocky Mountains than the Hollywood Hills.

BICYCLING

Just past the 31-mile mark, there is an overlook you don't want to miss. The view is of the San Fernando Valley—a spectacular, sprawling 20th-century development. Your view, at more that 3,400 feet, is as fine a terrestrial view of the valley as one can get. From here you have a mere 1.5-mile spin to the summit. Take a few minutes to have a bite and a drink.

The gradual grade of Santa Clara gives you a chance to settle into your rhythm. Stick it in the big ring and notch the chain down a few cogs. Given the chip-and-seal surface, don't go crazy on this descent.

Turn left at Little Tujunga Road and continue your descent. The road here twists and turns more tightly than Santa Clara did, and with the better pavement it makes more sense to let the bike run. Just as the 6.5-mile descent runs out, turn left on Placerita Canyon Road. Take a moment to pop your ears if they haven't popped themselves; you just dropped 2,000 vertical feet.

Placerita Canyon is kind of the cherry on top of this ride. It gradually gives up elevation, but it does so at a price. The road forces you over four rolling hills on its 4-mile run back to Sierra Highway. Traffic is a little heavier here; stay to the right even

though there isn't much shoulder.

Turn left on Sierra Highway and climb the short rise before you. This is officially your last hill of the day. Once at the top, you can begin turning over the big ring for the gradual downhill run back to your car.

Turn right on San Fernando. The final 5 miles back to the start are almost entirely downhill. With the later hour, take more care to watch the traffic around you. Keep an eye out for the historic Saugus Café on your left. As soon as you see it, work your way into the left lane for the left turn on Magic Mountain Parkway. Just 0.25 miles past the intersection, turn right up the ramp to enter the bike path. There is chain-link fence here; brake slightly before passing through the opening and rejoining the bike path. You have less than a mile before the final turn to the path that returns you to the town center.

After the Ride

Food is in order after this ride. In addition to several chain restaurants west of the parking structure, there is a mall with a diverse food court to the structure's east. Or you could consider driving back to the Saugus Café for some Wild West charm.

The view is of the San Fernando Valley— a spectacular, sprawling 20th-century development. Your view, at more that 3,400 feet, is as fine a terrestrial view of the valley as one can get.

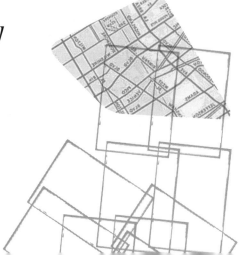

39 Glendora Mountain Road

AT A GLANCE

Length: 45 miles

Configuration: Loop

Difficulty: Difficult

Climbing: 4,500 feet

Maximum gradient: 10%

Scenery: Alpine environment and some city views

Exposure: Mornings and late afternoons can be overcast

Road traffic: Moderate

Road surface: Good

Riding time: 3.5 hours

Maps: Los Angeles County *Thomas Guide* pages 569, 509, 511, and 570

In Brief

Glendora Mountain Road is a challenging climb up into the San Gabriel Mountains at the far eastern edge of Los Angeles County. What distinguishes this road from other mountain roads is that it is closed to traffic. This is arguably the quietest, most peaceful climb a rider can make in the San Gabriel Mountains. After reaching the top, riders can attack the zigzagging road along the ridge, taking them to Mount Baldy, a small village that has a couple of restaurants, a lodge, a post office, and a fire department that resides in the shadow of Mount Baldy. Riders can either return by doubling back on their route or dropping into the Los Angeles basin.

Directions

From the intersection of I-605 and I-210, travel east on I-210. Exit at South Grand Avenue. Turn left at the bottom of the ramp, and drive 0.6 miles north on South Grand Avenue to East Alosta Avenue. Park in one of the parking lots in a commercial center here. There are a number of restaurants and stores in the area offering anything you may need before or after the ride.

Description

Unlike many rides in this guide, this one, because of its rather remote location, can be attempted almost any time of day without much concern for traffic. Bear in mind one thing: if you think you might want to take the flatter return route, leave early enough to avoid afternoon traffic. The bigger limitation on this ride is the season. Generally, the temperatures in the mountains are too cool to attempt this route from October to early March. The spur to Mount Baldy should really be attempted only during summer months.

Begin your ride by heading north on South Grand Avenue. Your first turn will be 1.25 miles up, at East Sierra Madre

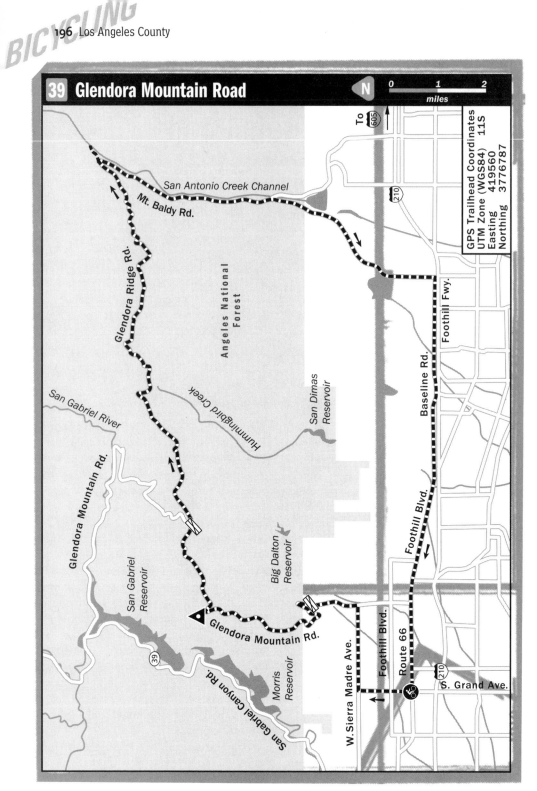

N

0   1   2
miles

GPS Trailhead Coordinates
UTM Zone (WGS84)   11S
Easting   419560
Northing   3776787

To 605

210

San Antonio Creek Channel

Mt. Baldy Rd.

Glendora Ridge Rd.

Angeles National Forest

San Gabriel River

Hummingbird Creek

San Dimas Reservoir

Baseline Rd.

Foothill Fwy.

Glendora Mountain Rd.

San Gabriel Reservoir

Big Dalton Reservoir

Glendora Mountain Rd.

Foothill Blvd.

39

Morris Reservoir

San Gabriel Canyon Rd.

W. Sierra Madre Ave.

Foothill Blvd.

Route 66

210

S. Grand Ave.

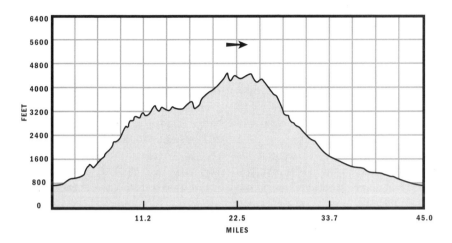

Avenue. Turn right on Sierra Madre and ride 2 miles to Glendora Mountain Road. Turn left on Glendora Mountain Road and begin climbing.

After passing Big Dalton Canyon Road, and just before you reach the gate closing the road, there is an area where it is possible to park, if you would prefer a more secluded and serene starting point for the ride. However, there are no restrooms or water here, and if you begin your ride after crossing the gate, you are forced to start the 8-mile climb with no warm-up whatsoever.

At the gate, dismount, step over the arm, and then lift your bike over. For the next 8 miles, the only time you will see any traffic is if there is a crew working to maintain the road following a springtime landslide. There is a very brief flat section to the first switchback, and then the road spirals skyward.

The climb from the gate to the top of the ridge ascends just more than 2,100 feet at an average gradient of 5 percent. The grade is surprisingly consistent on the climb; there are no big surprises.

The road features ten switchbacks in its first 3 miles after the gate. The constant change of direction and scenery is exciting enough to inspire a big effort through here. Following the last of the initial sequence of switchbacks, the road meanders up the ridgeline with a river's laziness—straight here, a little bend there—for the next 2.7 miles.

One of the most interesting aspects of the road in this section is the way it crosses

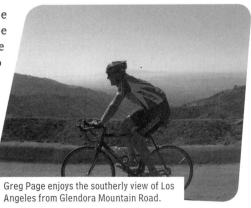

Greg Page enjoys the southerly view of Los Angeles from Glendora Mountain Road.

the ridgeline itself. At times your view will be to the southeast of the mountain, looking into Little Dalton Canyon; at other times, your view will be to the southwest and into San Gabriel Canyon. When you encounter the next right switchback, you'll notice a pullout on the left. This is Newman Point. You might consider stopping here to take in the view of the canyon below and back into the valley. Your elevation is 3,000 feet, and Morris Reservoir below you looks like a pond. Turning to the northwest, you will see the San Gabriel Dam and Reservoir. Newman Point is also significant because it gives you your first good views of the interior of the San Gabriel range. You will be able to see 10,000-foot Mount San Antonio (also known as Old Baldy) piercing the sky, its peak painted gray with rocks and scree.

From Newman Point to the top of the climb, you ride another 2.3 miles. As you head away from Newman Point, your view will continue to be to the north for roughly a mile, whereupon the road veers back to the southern side of the ridge, giving you a dramatic view of the city—provided the haze isn't too bad.

Following a brief descent to Horse Canyon Saddle, you reach the gate at the top of Glendora Mountain Road. Dismount and step over the gate. At this point, Glendora Mountain Road turns left and descends toward San Gabriel Canyon. Stay to the right on Glendora Ridge Road.

Glendora Ridge Road is unusual among the roads traversing the San Gabriel Mountains in that it follows a ridgeline for the whole of its path. Most roads in the San Gabriels were paved to cross the range from north to south, or to ascend to one of the peaks. The other notable exception is Angeles Forest Highway, which you can ride on the Mount Wilson Loop (page 200).

The 11.6-mile Glendora Ridge Road cuts a largely east–west route well within the San Gabriels. You are rarely out of view of Mount San Antonio. Initially, it sawtooths its way up and down the edge of the ridge, but that changes rather dramatically at Peacock Saddle. The last four hills have limited your altitude to between 3,200 and 3,600 feet of elevation. Peacock Saddle (at 3,390 feet) comes 4.6 miles after you begin Glendora Ridge Road. The climb is 3.6 miles long and reaches an altitude of 4,575 feet, gaining 1,185 feet on an average gradient of 6 percent. The climb can be difficult to judge, though. With more than a dozen switchbacks, the views are great, but you can't see the top until you're practically there.

The sawtoothing resumes at the top for 2.7 miles before making a short (0.9-mile, 300-foot) drop to the village of Mount Baldy. Technically, the town is in San Bernardino County, but this is the only portion of the ride that is. In town (it's not much of a town, though), there are two restaurants and a soda machine. Should you choose to do this ride on a weekday, it is possible the restaurants will be closed; you can find water at a faucet to the left of the fountain at the entrance to the Buckhorn Lodge.

At this point, you can choose an optional climb. If you're interested in pursuing it, make sure you are on top of your climbing form and have plenty of food. The out-and-back to Mount Baldy is 14 miles—that's another 7 miles of climbing with 3,500 feet of elevation gain. Sea-level dwellers will enjoy the thin air at the top; the climb reaches 7,800 feet. This is likely the most difficult sustained climb in Southern California—the 7-mile ascent averages a brutal 9.5 percent.

Whether you choose to tackle the bonus climb or not, there are two possible return routes from the village of Mount Baldy. You can either double back on the route you took to the village, or you can drop back into the valley on Mount Baldy Road and take a much flatter route back. If you're feeling saucy, take Glendora Ridge Road back to Glendora Mountain Road and descend from there. The terrain is more fun in this direction, and there's only another 1,000 feet of climbing on the way back.

Should you prefer an easier, less technical ride back, you can simply ride down Mount Baldy Road. Although this descent doesn't have all the twists and bends of Glendora Mountain Road, it is still a quick descent, and your speed can easily climb upward of 40 mph.

The descent will take you from about 4,200 feet to 1,600 feet of elevation before you encounter significant turns. First, Mount Baldy will merge with North Mills Avenue. Mills will continue to descend, though more gently now. Turn right at West Baseline Road. You will ride 4.7 miles on Baseline. There is a wide shoulder here, and very often there is a bike lane. Despite the traffic, this road isn't nerve wracking.

At Foothill Boulevard, turn right. Foothill is also the historic Route 66, and though many roads comprise that famed highway, there is a section of Foothill that is one of the few places where the road is actually labeled Route 66. Take Foothill 4.8 miles to Grand Avenue, turn right, and pull back into the parking lot.

After the Ride
Glendora is a suburb and isn't the most fascinating tourist mecca. There are, however, plenty of enjoyable restaurants nearby to fuel up. And frankly, if you took in Mount Baldy, you probably won't be interested in much more than a big meal.

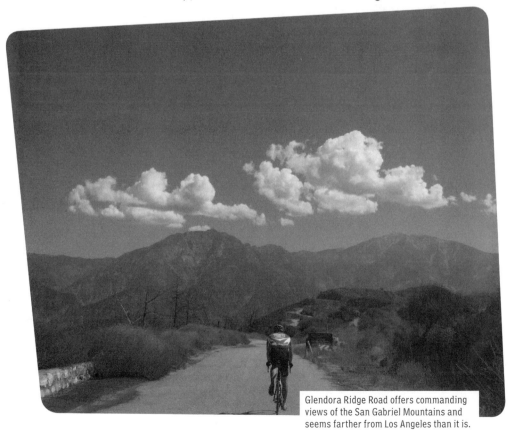

Glendora Ridge Road offers commanding views of the San Gabriel Mountains and seems farther from Los Angeles than it is.

40 Mount Wilson Loop

AT A GLANCE

Length: 50 miles

Configuration: Loop

Difficulty: Difficult

Climbing: 4,700 feet

Maximum gradient: 9%

Scenery: Dense forest, rocky cliffs, incredible views of Los Angeles

Exposure: Severe; the only shade comes when riding in the shadow of a mountain

Road traffic: Moderate

Road surface: Good to excellent

Riding time: 4.5 hours

Maps: Los Angeles County *Thomas Guide* pages 534, 504, 503, 4643, 4645, 505, and 535

In Brief

Mount Wilson may be one of the more modest peaks in the San Gabriel range, but its location gives it an unbeatable view of the city. The loop is almost perfectly binary: you climb, then you descend. You will be amazed at how remote much of the ride seems despite its proximity to the metropolis.

Directions

From the interchange of I-5 and I-110, drive north 2 miles on I-5 to the exit for CA 2. Take CA 2 north 8 miles and exit at Foothill Boulevard. Turn left on Foothill and drive 1.4 miles northwest. Just after you pass Rosemont Drive, there is a large commercial development on the right. Pull in there to park.

Description

Because this ride involves so much climbing, it is important that you arrive prepared.

Aside from training on some climbs that last more than 20 minutes at a stretch, you would do well to hone your descending skills; you will spend more than a half-hour descending. Being comfortable on a twisty road at 35 mph will make this ride much more enjoyable. Technical concerns are largely limited to gearing. Provided the rest of your equipment is in proper working order, just make sure you have gearing low enough for the descent. The bare minimum for this ride is 39 x 25. If you don't consider yourself a strong climber, consider a 27t cog, a compact crank, or a triple. You may want to bring along arm warmers and a vest for the descent.

From the parking lot, turn right onto Foothill Boulevard and ride northwest. Initially, the road is flat, but that quickly changes when you encounter a steady 3-percent incline. Foothill is a large boulevard, but it has a wide shoulder that can easily accommodate a cyclist. Like many

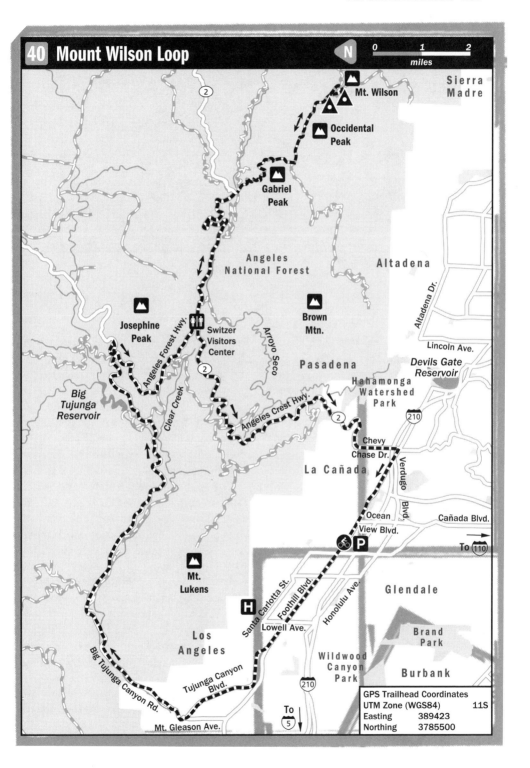

40 **Mount Wilson Loop**

Sierra Madre

Mt. Wilson

Occidental Peak

Gabriel Peak

Angeles National Forest

Altadena

Josephine Peak

Switzer Visitors Center

Brown Mtn.

Angeles Forest Hwy.

Clear Creek

Arroyo Seco

Pasadena

Hahamonga Watershed Park

Devils Gate Reservoir

Altadena Dr.

Lincoln Ave.

Big Tujunga Reservoir

Angeles Crest Hwy.

210

Chevy Chase Dr.

La Cañada

Verdugo Blvd.

Cañada Blvd.

Ocean View Blvd.

To 110

Mt. Lukens

H

Santa Carlotta St.

Foothill Blvd.

Honolulu Ave.

Lowell Ave.

Glendale

Brand Park

Big Tujunga Canyon Rd.

Los Angeles

Tujunga Canyon Blvd.

210

Wildwood Canyon Park

Burbank

Mt. Gleason Ave.

To 5

GPS Trailhead Coordinates
UTM Zone (WGS84)   11S
Easting   389423
Northing   3785500

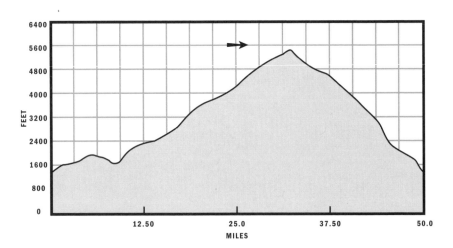

rides in this guide, this is a loop that is best attempted early on a weekend day. If you wish to do this on a weekday, leave especially early—before rush hour begins. On weekend mornings, there are almost no parked cars on the roadside, so you generally have the whole shoulder between you and what little traffic there is.

Your first turn comes 2.8 miles into the ride. Turn right on Tujunga Canyon Boulevard. Do not make the mistake of turning right onto Tujunga Canyon *Place*, which comes just 100 meters sooner.

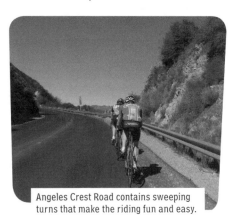
Angeles Crest Road contains sweeping turns that make the riding fun and easy.

Tujunga Canyon Boulevard is a residential street that takes you away from the traffic and development of Foothill. No matter how good your timing is, this route will be quieter and more peaceful than Foothill Boulevard. Your turn onto Tujunga Canyon Boulevard is slight; it is more of a fork in the road than the 90-degree turn that Tujunga Canyon Place is.

The road will immediately bend left to parallel Foothill and then curl right to head more directly north toward the canyon. Most of this residential section will descend toward the big climb. Simply watch the signs for Tujunga Canyon, and you will negotiate each of the bends without getting lost. Turn left onto Plainview Avenue at 5.1 miles. Less than a half-mile later, turn right on Mount Gleason Avenue. This road bends a bit; following a switchback right and a bend to the left, Mount Gleason intersects Big Tujunga Canyon. Turn right and enjoy the brief flat as best you can; it's likely you will encounter a headwind caused by the temperature differential between the warmer air of the valley and the cooler air in the mountains.

The mountain roads that dominate this ride are not heavily trafficked. Most vehicles are those of motorcyclists out enjoying the roads just like you, though perhaps at slightly higher speeds.

Your easy pedaling will last exactly a mile. At this point, 7 miles into your route, abandon all hope. OK, maybe that's a little severe; prepare yourself for some sustained climbing. The road ascends incessantly for the next 9.8 miles, rising more than 1,700 vertical feet, making it one of a handful of climbs longer than 5 miles that averages more than a 3-percent gradient (3.3, in this case). The road takes a very direct route up into the canyon initially. It's not until 13.5 miles into the ride that Big Tujunga Canyon begins to writhe through more-traditional alpine switchbacks. Once it does, though, the views will evolve constantly with each new bend.

Passing 15 miles, look off to your left and down the hillside you will see Big Tujunga Reservoir. You are close to your next turn. At 16.8 miles, Big Tujunga Canyon encounters Angeles Forest Highway. Turn right on Angeles Forest. The road cuts a lazy arcing path around Josephine Peak, rising to a height of 5,558 feet above sea level. With the exception of one short downhill, the road continues to gently climb for the next 3.8 miles, until it intersects Angeles Crest Highway (also known as CA 2—which you drove on to get to the ride's start).

The Switzer Visitor Center, which has information on the area in the form of maps and books, plus traveler's advisories, is at the intersection of Angeles Forest and Angeles Crest. If you need a bathroom break or more water, this is your first big chance since you began climbing Big Tujunga Canyon. The water fountain is on the right side of the visitor center as you face the entrance.

From the parking lot, turn right onto

The loop is almost perfectly binary: you climb, then you descend. You will be amazed at how remote much of the ride seems despite its proximity to the metropolis.

Angeles Crest. After a brief drop that helps you build some momentum, the climbing resumes. Over the next 3.8 miles, Angeles Crest rises some 1,100 feet, averaging 5.5 percent. Initially, the road winds slightly, carving a gentle serpentine, but then you pedal through a sequence of four switchbacks just before reaching the ranger's station at Red Box. There is a water fountain on the right side of the road opposite the parking lot, and there are bathrooms in the parking lot. Take a moment to pull into the parking area to look out on the mountains and forest as they spread to the east.

Turn right on Mount Wilson Highway. The 5.3-mile climb rises just more than 1,000 feet for an average gradient of nearly 4 percent. Some riders may begin to feel the first effects of the altitude, noticing they can't keep their speed up, despite maintaining a high heart rate. You will get two solid opportunities to recover on brief flats and even one very brief downhill.

Of all the roads you encounter on the ride, this one will have the least traffic. Because it is a road to nowhere, the only cars you'll see will be of people heading to the top of Mount Wilson for a look around. Mount Wilson Highway cuts its way along the north side of Mount Wilson, so your ride up looks east, north, and west, but not south. Across the San Gabriel Wilderness, you can see Angeles Crest make its way along the spine of the San Gabriel range. Filling the valley below is a diverse forest composed of oaks, maples, and pines, among others.

Mount Wilson hosts a number of television and radio antennae. You will be able to gauge your progress by watching the ridgeline from which they emerge. Finally, you'll pass a stand of trees, and suddenly the Los Angeles basin will sprawl before you. The view is as startling as it is breathtaking. A small loop of asphalt encircles much of the antennae installation. As you wind the counterclockwise loop, you will be able to view everything from the coast and the Palos Verdes Peninsula to Orange County, the Santa Monica Mountains, the Verdugo and Hollywood Hills, and clear into Riverside County. And rising from the middle of it is downtown Los Angeles and its skyscrapers, at once impressive and miniscule. In a city full of amazing sights, this is one not to miss.

Want to hear the great news? Your ride back to the car requires almost no effort. There's a small rise on the way down Mount Wilson, and a half-mile climb to get to the Switzer Visitor Center, but no other challenges until you reach Foothill Boulevard.

When you pass the visitor center, continue straight on Angeles Crest rather than turning right on Angeles Forest. The road will run flat for a little more than a mile before resuming its descent. The pavement is new here, and the countertop-smooth surface makes for great— and safe—descending. The bends, twists, and turns of Angeles Crest are based on large, lazy arcs. These, combined with a fairly gentle grade, allow you to slalom the two dozen switchbacks of the descent with ease. Your only cause for concern will be cars that pass you as they descend—the large-radius turns permit them to speed down at impressive, if slightly suicidal, speeds; watch your back so you know when to pull to the right.

Following a final sweeping left, Angeles Crest straightens for its run straight downhill to Foothill. This is the steepest section of the descent, and it is where you need to be most careful because there are cars pulling into the road from side streets and driveways.

Turn right on Foothill. At this point, you are 2.5 miles from your car. You'll climb a bit more, and then the road will remain fairly flat back to the parking lot. Despite the later hour, the wide lane should give you plenty of room to feel safe in the traffic.

After the Ride

The commercial development where you parked has several restaurants to sate your postachievement appetite. If you feel up for a walk and haven't already visited Descanso Gardens, enjoy a mellow afternoon there.

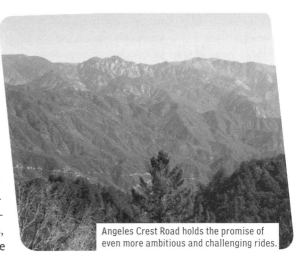
Angeles Crest Road holds the promise of even more ambitious and challenging rides.

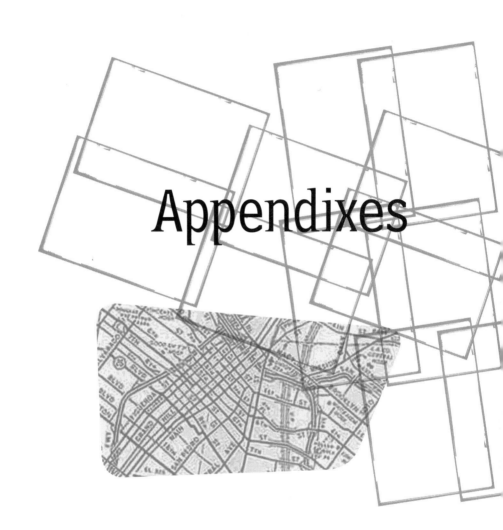

Appendixes

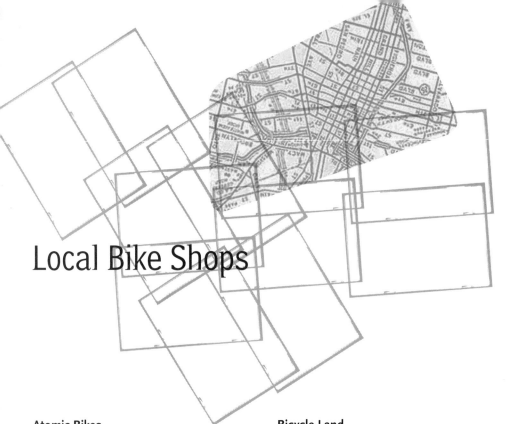

Local Bike Shops

Atomic Bikes
www.atomicbikes.com
14360 Telegraph Road
Whittier, CA 90604
(562) 944-4696

Aviation Cyclery
1075 North Aviation Boulevard
Manhattan Beach, CA 90266
(310) 372-1910
aviationcycle@aol.com

Beach Cities Cycle
219 Pacific Coast Highway
Hermosa Beach, CA 90254
(310) 318-6030

Bellflower Bicycles
16442 Woodruff Avenue
Bellflower, CA 90706
(562) 867-2306

Bicycle Land
422 North Glendale Avenue
Glendale, CA 91206
(818) 242-6906

The Bike Connection
13711 Ventura Boulevard
Sherman Oaks, CA 91423
(818) 995-5788

Bike Land Cypress
5530 Lincoln Avenue
Cypress, CA 90630
(714) 995-6541

The Bike Palace
www.thebikepalace.com
1600-B South Pacific Avenue
San Pedro, CA 90731-4105
(310) 832-1966

Bike Rite
11126 1/2 Ramona Boulevard
El Monte, CA 91731
(626) 444-3981

The Bike Shop
430 Pier Ave
Hermosa Beach, CA 90254
(310) 376-2914

Bikecology
9006 West Pico Boulevard
Los Angeles, CA 90035-1310
(310) 278-0915
bikecologyla@yahoo.com

Bikecology
4051 Lincoln Boulevard
Marina Del Ray, CA 90292
(310) 821-0766

Bikecology
2355 Sepulveda Boulevard
Torrance, CA 90501
(310) 320-1417

Bill Rons Bicycles
807 Torrance Boulevard
Redondo Beach, CA 90277-3529
(310) 540-2080
billronbikes@earthlink.net

Boardwalk Skates
201 1/2 Ocean Front Walk
Venice, CA 90291
(310) 450-6634

Budget Pro Bikes
2750 Colorado Boulevard
Eagle Rock, CA 90041-0000
(323) 254-4160

Buena Park Bicycle Co.
www.buenaparkbicycle.com
6042 Beach Boulevard
Buena Park, CA 90621
(714) 521-8120
info@fullertonbicycle.com

Burbank Bike Shop
4400 West Victory Boulevard
Burbank, CA 91505-1335
(818) 848-6177

California Cycle Sport
6759 Carson Street
Lakewood, CA 90713-3241
(562) 425-0704

Carson Schwinn
251 East Carson Street
Carson, CA 90745-2705
(310) 549-3939

Corbin's Redondo Bicycle
607 South Pacific Coast Highway
Redondo Beach, CA 90277-4222
(310) 543-3226

Custom Bicycle Sales Inc.
18424 1/2 Ventura Boulevard
Tarzana, CA 91356-4256
(818) 344-2806

Cycleworx
www.cycleworxla.com
5003 York Boulevard
Los Angeles, CA 90042
(323) 259-3131
info@cycleworxla.com

Cycling Concepts
www.cyclingconcepts.net
12148 South Street
Artesia, CA 90701
(562) 865-9571
cyclingconcepts@verizon.net

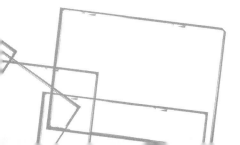

BICYCLING

Cycology
www.cycologybikes.com
14456 Ventura Boulevard
Sherman Oaks, CA 91423-2607
(818) 986-2544
tony@cycologybikes.com

Cynergy
www.cynergycycles.com
2300 Santa Monica Boulevard
Santa Monica, CA 90404
customerservice@cynergycycles.com

Europa Bicycle Center
6217 Van Nuys Boulevard
Van Nuys, CA 91401-2710
(818) 989-2453

G's Cyclery and Wheels
6713 Greenleaf Avenue
Whittier, CA 90601
(562) 698-9426

Glendale Cyclery
1250 West Glen Oaks Boulevard, Suite A
Glendale, CA 91201-2268
(818) 246-5551
glendalecycle@earthlink.net

H & S Bicycles
2316 West Victory Boulevard
Burbank CA 91506
(818) 848-8551
hsbikes@yahoo.com

Helen's Cycles
www.helenscycles.com
1570 #C Rosencrans
Manhattan Beach, CA 90266
(310) 643-9140

Helen's Cycles
www.helenscycles.com
2501 Broadway Street
Santa Monica, CA 90404-3045
(310) 829-1836

Helen's Cycles
www.helenscycles.com
2472 Lincoln Boulevard
Venice, CA 90291-5041
(310) 306-7843

Helen's Cycles
www.helenscycles.com
1071 Gayley Avenue
Westwood, CA 90024-3401
(310) 208-8988

I. Martin Imports
www.imartin.com
8330 Beverly Boulevard
Los Angeles, CA 90048
(323) 653-6900
info@imartin.com

Jax Bicycle Center
www.jaxbicycles.com
3000 North Bellflower Boulevard
Long Beach, CA 90808
(562) 421-4646

Jones Bicycles
www.jonesbicycles.com
5332 East 2nd Street
Long Beach, CA 90803-5332
(562) 434-0343
info@jonesbicycles.com

Jones Bicycles
2523 Huntington Drive
San Marino, CA 91108-2603
(626) 793-4227
ferretboy@sbcglobal.net

La Habra Cyclery
451 North Harbor Boulevard
La Habra, CA 90631
(562) 691-7118
raceturtle@aol.com

Martins Bike Shop
6067 East Olympic Boulevard
Los Angeles, CA 90022
(323) 832-5304

Montrose Bike Shop
www.montrosebike.com
2501 Honolulu Avenue
Montrose, CA 91020-1805
(818) 249-3993

Pasadena Cyclery
www.pasadenacyclery.com
1670 East Walnut Street
Pasadena, CA 91106-1619
(626) 584-6391

Pats 605 Cyclery Inc.
12310 Studebaker Road
Norwalk, CA 90650

PV Bicycle Center
www.pvbike.com
714 Deep Valley Drive
Rolling Hills Estates, CA 90274
(310) 377-7441

Reseda Bikes
7056 Reseda Boulevard
Reseda, CA 91335-4208
(818) 345-8844

Russells Bicycles
8027 East Firestone
Downey, CA 90241
(562) 862-4837

Safety Cycle
1014 North Western Avenue
Los Angeles, CA 90029-2310
(323) 464-5765

Sea Mist Rental
1619 Ocean
Santa Monica, CA 90401
(310) 395-7076
trm@pacificnet.net

Smith's Cycle
www.smithscycle.com
2073 Pacific Coast Highway
Lomita, CA 90717
(310) 326-0617
sales@smithscycle.com

Stan's Monrovia Bikes
800 South Myrtle Avenue
Monrovia, CA 91016
(626) 357-0020

Universal Cycles, Inc.
3717 Cahuenga Boulevard
Studio City, CA 91604-3504
(818) 980-7456
universal-Cycles@earthlink.net

Van's Cyclery
11407 Victory Boulevard
North Hollywood, CA 91606-3615
(818) 760-6960

Wheel World
www.wheelworld.com
4051 Sepulveda Boulevard
Culver City, CA 90230-4609
(310) 391-5251

Wheel World
www.wheelworld.com
22718 Ventura Boulevard
Woodland Hills, CA 91364
(818) 224-2044
sales@wheelworld.com

Whittier Cyclery
10316 Santa Gertrudes
Whittier, CA 90603
(562) 947-1214

Willy's Bike
11968 Foothill Boulevard
Lake View Terrace, CA 91342-7101
(818) 896-4249
w6101865@msn.com

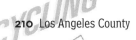

Bike Clubs
in Los Angeles County

Club	Web Site	Community
LA Wheelmen	www.lawheelmen.org	Los Angeles
South Bay Wheelmen	www.sbwheelmen.org	Redondo Beach
Foothill Cycle Club	www.foothillcycle.org	Pasadena
San Fernando Valley Bicycle Club	www.sfvbc.org	Los Angeles
LaGrange	www.lagrange.org	Westwood
Dockriders Cycling Club	www.dockriders.com	Los Angeles
West LA Cycling Club	www.wlacyclingclub.com	Los Angeles
Cynergy Cycles	www.cynergycycles.com	Santa Monica
Peninsula Cycle Club	www.peninsulacc.org	San Pedro
Santa Clarita Velo	www.santaclaritavelo.com	Santa Clarita
Lightning Velo	www.lightningvelo.org	Long Beach
Covina Cycle Club	www.covinacycleclub.org	Covina
Velo Allegro	www.veloallegro.org	Long Beach
Pasadena Athletic Association Cycling Club	www.paacycling.org	Pasadena
Shifting Gears	www.shiftinggearscycling.com	Santa Monica
Team Martini	www.teammartini.net	Santa Monica
Beverly Hills Spokesmen	sports.groups.yahoo.com/ group/beverlyhillsspokesmen/	Beverly Hills
Calvary Cycling Association	www.calvarygs.org/calvary/ cycling/index.htm	Diamond Bar

Advocacy Organizations

Los Angeles County Bicycle Coalition	www.labike.org	Los Angeles
California Association of Bicycling Organizations	www.cabobike.org	Los Angeles

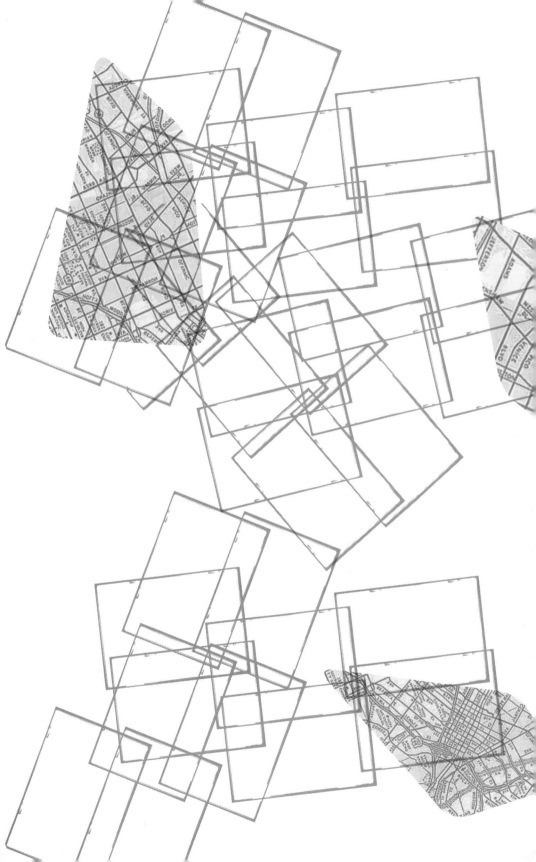

Regularly Recurring Group Rides

All rides are free, but some clubs may require you to sign a liability waiver form.

SPONSORING CLUB/RIDE NAME	CITY	START LOCATION
High Desert Cyclists	Acton	Bicycle John's 33330 Santiago Rd.
Bud's Ride	Claremont	2nd St. at Yale Ave.
Covina Cycle Club	Covina	Covina Park
Diamond Bar Cyclery	Diamond Bar	1125 S. Grand Ave.
Calvary Cycling Association	Diamond Bar	22324 Golden Springs Dr.
High Desert Cyclists	Lancaster	Gil's Bike Shop 43791 N. 15th St. W.
Local	Lancaster	20th W. at Avenue L
Team Block	Lancaster	Quartz Hill High School
Team Block	Lancaster	Block Shop 42217 12th St. W.
Team Block	Lancaster	Block Shop 42217 12th St. W.
6th Street Crit	Lancaster	Block Shop 42217 12th S.W.
Lightning Velo	Long Beach	El Dorado Park W., 2800 Studebaker
Lightning Velo	Long Beach	El Dorado Park W., 2800 Studebaker
Velo Allegro	Long Beach	Long Beach Marina at Westminster
Velo Allegro	Long Beach	Long Beach Marina at Westminster
Velo Allegro	Long Beach	Long Beach Marina at Westminster
Velo Allegro	Long Beach	Long Beach Marina at Westminster
Velo Allegro	Long Beach	Long Beach Marina at Westminster
Velo Allegro	Long Beach	Long Beach Marina at Westminster
Velo Allegro	Long Beach	Long Beach Marina at Westminster
Hughes Park	Long Beach	S. Santa Fe Ave. at W. Carson St.
West LA Cycling Club	Los Angeles	Varies
Shifting Gears Cycling Club	Los Feliz	Hillhurst at Ambrose
The Kettle Ride	Manhattan Beach	Manhattan Beach Blvd. at Highland Ave.
Holiday Ride	Manhattan Beach	Manhattan Beach Blvd. at Highland Ave

TIME	DAY	PACE	COURSE	MILEAGE	INFO
8:00 a.m.	2nd and 4th Saturday	Varies	Varies	20–60	www.highdesertcyclists.com
5:30 p.m.	Wednesday	Fast	Hills	25–30	www.socalcycling.com
8:00 a.m.	Saturday	Varies	Varies	26–62	www.covinacycleclub.org
7:30 a.m.	Saturday	Varies	Varies	Varies	www.diamondbarcyclery.com
9:00 a.m.	Saturday	Varies	Varies	15–30	www.calvarygs.org/calvary/cycling
Varies	1st and 3rd Saturday	Varies	Varies	Varies	www.highdesertcyclists.com
8:00 a.m.	Sat./Sun.	Fast	Varies	45–65	www.highdesertcyclists.com
6:00 a.m.	Thursday	Moderate	Flat	60	www.teamblock.com
7:00 a.m.	Saturday	Fast	Hills	40	www.teamblock.com
7:00 a.m.	Sunday	Fast	Hills	50	www.teamblock.com
7:00 p.m.	Mon./Wed.	Varies	Flat	1–2 hours	www.teamblock.com
7:30 a.m.	Saturday	Easy to fast	Mostly flat	40	lightningvelo.org
7:30 a.m.	Sunday	Fast	Varies	51–72	lightningvelo.org
7:00 a.m.	Monday	Easy	Varies	Varies	www.veloallegro.org
6:30 a.m.	Tuesday	Intervals	Varies	Varies	www.veloallegro.org
7:00 a.m.	Wednesday	Tempo	Varies	Varies	www.veloallegro.org
7:00 a.m.	Thursday	Fast	Varies	Varies	www.veloallegro.org
7:00 a.m.	Friday	Sprints	Varies	Varies	www.veloallegro.org
7:30 a.m.	Saturday	Fast	Mostly flat	30	www.veloallegro.org
7:30 a.m.	Sunday	Fast	Varies	Varies	www.veloallegro.org
7:30 p.m.	Thursday	Fast	Flat	29	www.socalcycling.com
Varies	Sat./Sun.	Easy	Mostly flat	25	www.wlacyclingclub.com
6:45 a.m.	Thursday	Easy	Hills	15	www.shiftinggearcycling.com
7:00 a.m.	Sunday	Fast	Flat or hills	50–70	www.southbaywheelmen.org
8:00 a.m.	National holidays*	Moderate	Flat w/one hill	50–55	www.southbaywheelmen.org

* All national holidays--New Year's, Memorial Day, 4th of July, Labor Day, Thanksgiving, Christmas
** 8:00 a.m. in the winter   **** 8:30 a.m. from November to April*

SPONSORING CLUB/RIDE NAME	CITY	START LOCATION
Weed Whackers	Manhattan Beach	Beach Bike Path at Rosecrans
Dock Riders	Marina Del Rey	Dock 52 Fiji Way
Dock Riders	Marina Del Rey	Dock 52 Fiji Way
San Fernando Valley Bicycle Club	Northridge	Nordhoff at Etiwanda
Doctor's Ride	Palos Verdes Estates	276 Palos Verdes Dr. W.
Weed Whackers	Palos Verdes Estates	276 Palos Verdes Dr. W.
Foothill Cycle Club	Pasadena	Diamond and El Centro
Foothill Cycle Club	Pasadena	Huntington at Rosemead
Foothill Cycle Club	Pasadena	Victory Park
Peninsula Cycle Club	Rancho Palos Verdes	Palos Verdes Dr. N. at Palos Verdes Dr. E.
Easy Riser	Redondo Beach	Catalina Coffee Co. 126 Catalina Ave.
South Bay Wheelmen	Redondo Beach	Torrance at Broadway
Beach Cities Cycling Club	Redondo Beach	Varies
Foothill Cycle Club	San Gabriel Valley	Varies
Peninsula Cycle Club	San Pedro	Bike Palace 1600-B S. Pacific Ave.
Santa Clarita Velo	Santa Clarita	Performance Cyclery 26067 Bouquet Canyon Rd.
Heritage Park	Santa Fe Springs	Heritage Park Dr. at Telegraph Rd.
La Grange	Santa Monica	26th at San Vicente
La Grange	Santa Monica	26th at San Vicente
La Grange	Santa Monica	26th at San Vicente
La Grange	Santa Monica	26th at San Vicente
Local	Santa Monica	Ocean at San Vicente
Local	Santa Monica	Ocean at San Vicente
Shifting Gears Cycling Club	Santa Monica	Peet's Coffee 2439 Main St.
Shifting Gears Cycling Club	Santa Monica	Varies
Tour of Sierra Madre	Sierra Madre	2563 E. Colorado Blvd.
Telo	Torrance	Kashiwa at Telo

TIME	DAY	PACE	COURSE	MILEAGE	INFO
9:00 a.m.	Tuesday	Moderate	Varies	50–60	www.southbaywheelmen.org
8:00 a.m.	Saturday	Varies	Varies	40–50	www.dockriders.com
8:15 a.m.	Sunday	Varies	Varies	40–50	www.dockriders.com
8:00 a.m.	Sat./Sun./ Mon./Wed.	Varies	Varies	25–90	sfvbc.org
7:00 a.m.	Saturday	Moderate	Hills	35–50	www.southbaywheelmen.org
9:30 a.m.	Thursday	Moderate	Hills	40–50	www.southbaywheelmen.org
9:00 a.m.	Tuesday	Moderate	Hills	25	www.foothillcycle.org
9:00 a.m.	Wednesday	Moderate	Flat	30	www.foothillcycle.org
8:00 a.m.***	Sunday	Fast	Varies	20–60	www.foothillcycle.org
9:00 a.m.	Tuesday	Moderate	Hills		www.peninsulacc.org
9:30 a.m.	Saturday	Easy	Beginners	20–30	www.southbaywheelmen.org
9:00 a.m.	Sunday	Moderate	Hills	30–40	www.southbaywheelmen.org
7:30 or 9:00 a.m.	Sat./Sun.	Easy to moderate	Varies	20–60	www.beachcitiescycling.com
Varies	Saturday	Varies	Varies	20–60	www.foothillcycle.org
7:00 a.m.	Saturday	Moderate	Hills		www.peninsulacc.org
7:00 a.m.**	Sat./Sun.	Moderate to fast	Varies	20-80	www.santaclaritavelo.com
8:00 p.m.	Tuesday	Fast	Flat	24	www.socalcycling.com
6:30 a.m.	Tuesday	Fast	Flat	29	www.lagrange.org
6:30 a.m.	Wednesday	Moderate	Hills	27	www.lagrange.org
6:30 a.m.	Thursday	Fast	Hills	29	www.lagrange.org
6:30 a.m.	Friday	Easy	Recovery	25	www.lagrange.org
8:00 a.m.	Saturday	Varies	Varies	Varies	www.lagrange.org
8:00 a.m.	Sunday	Varies	Varies	Varies	www.lagrange.org
6:30 a.m.	Tuesday	Varies	Flat	15	www.shiftinggearcycling.com
8:30 a.m.	Sunday	Easy	Varies	20-75	www.shiftinggearcycling.com
6:00 p.m.	Wednesday	Moderate to fast	Hills	30	www.socalcycling.com
6:00 p.m.	Tuesday	Fast	Flat	1 hour	www.southbaywheelmen.org

Index

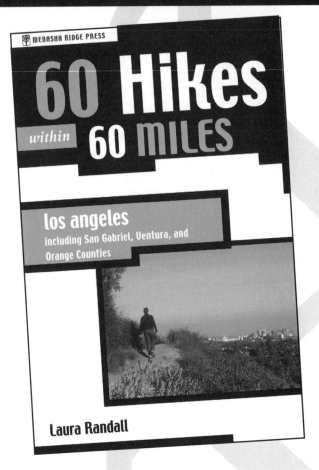

DEAR CUSTOMERS AND FRIENDS,

SUPPORTING YOUR INTEREST IN OUTDOOR ADVENTURE, travel, and an active lifestyle is central to our operations, from the authors we choose to the locations we detail to the way we design our books. Menasha Ridge Press was incorporated in 1982 by a group of veteran outdoorsmen and professional outfitters. For 25 years now, we've specialized in creating books that benefit the outdoors enthusiast.

Almost immediately, Menasha Ridge Press earned a reputation for revolutionizing outdoors- and travel-guidebook publishing. For such activities as canoeing, kayaking, hiking, backpacking, and mountain biking, we established new standards of quality that transformed the whole genre, resulting in outdoor-recreation guides of great sophistication and solid content. Menasha Ridge continues to be outdoor publishing's greatest innovator.

The folks at Menasha Ridge Press are as at home on a white-water river or mountain trail as they are editing a manuscript. The books we build for you are the best they can be, because we're responding to your needs. Plus, we use and depend on them ourselves.

We look forward to seeing you on the river or the trail. If you'd like to contact us directly, join in at www.trekalong.com or visit us at www.menasharidge.com. We thank you for your interest in our books and the natural world around us all.

SAFE TRAVELS,

Bob Sehlinger

BOB SEHLINGER
PUBLISHER

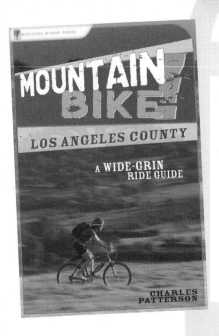
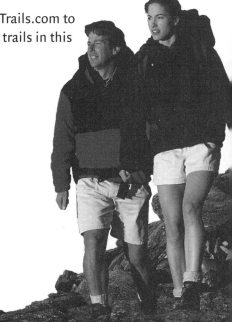
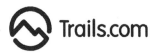